Love and Anger
Essays on AIDS, Activism, and Politics

Love and Anger
Essays on AIDS, Activism, and Politics

Peter F. Cohen

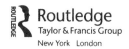
Routledge
Taylor & Francis Group
New York   London

First published by

Harrington Park Press, an imprint of The Haworth Press, Inc., 10 Alice Street, Binghamton, NY 13904-1580

This edition published 2013 by Routledge

Routledge   Routledge
Taylor & Francis Group   Taylor & Francis Group
711 Third Avenue   2 Park Square, Milton Park
New York, NY 10017   Abingdon, Oxon OX14 4RN

Routledge is an imprint of the Taylor & Francis Group, an informa business

Material from *People in Trouble* by Sarah Schulman, © 1990 by Sarah Schulman, is used with permission from Dutton Signet, a division of Penguin Books USA Inc.

Material from *The Normal Heart* by Larry Kramer, © 1985 by Larry Kramer, is used with permission from Dutton Signet, a division of Penguin Books USA Inc.

Material from *Angels in America, Part Two: Perestroika* by Tony Kushner, © 1994 by Tony Kushner, is used with permission from Theatre Communications Group.

Material from *Afterlife* by Paul Monette, © 1990 by Paul Monette, is used with permission from Crown Publishers.

Cover design by Monica L. Seifert.

Cover photo used by permission of Duncan A. Smith.

The Library of Congress has cataloged the hardcover edition of this book as:

Cohen, Peter F. (Peter Franzblau)
    Love and anger : essays on AIDS, activism, and politics / Peter F. Cohen.
        p.   cm.
    Includes bibliographical references and index.
    ISBN 0-7890-0455-0 (alk. paper).
    1. AIDS (Disease)—Political aspects—United States. 2. ACT UP (Organization). I. Title.
RA644.A25C58 1998
362.1'969792'00973—dc21   97-51814
                                                                                  CIP

ISBN 1-56023-930-1 (pbk.)

CONTENTS

ABOUT THE AUTHOR

Peter F. Cohen is a former member of ACT UP, the AIDS Coalition to Unleash Power. He holds a doctoral degree in American Studies, with a speciality in gay and lesbian studies. His articles have appeared in the *Journal of the History of Sexuality* and the *Hemingway Review.* Mr. Cohen can be reached via the Internet at peterfcohen@post.harvard.edu.

Acknowledgments

I am extremely indebted to a number of people for their assistance in the completion of this book. *Love and Anger* began as my PhD dissertation at Brown University and would not exist without the help and support of my dissertation committee: David Savran, Susan Smulyan, and Neil Lazarus. Jessica Shubow, Jennifer Ting, Melani McAlister, and Karin Cope offered early comments on the dissertation proposal. Duncan A. Smith, Kathy Franz, Vernon Rosario, Timothy Engels, Sarah Schulman, Stephen Shapiro, Miriam Reumann, Lisa Duggan, Maxine Wolfe, Daniel Cavicchi, Jane Gerhard, Bob Lederer, Robert Mack, Janice Okoomian, and J.P. Gownder read and commented on sections of the manuscript. Kristen Farmelant and Daniel Cavicchi assisted me in setting up a workshop on conducting oral histories, at which Paul Buhle was an additional speaker.

The Swearer Center for Public Service at Brown University provided me with a small grant to offset costs related to my fieldwork. Arthur Mandel and Claudia Nahson provided hospitality and theater company during my many trips to New York. Maxine Wolfe and David Román kindly allowed me to read unpublished manuscripts of theirs. My thinking in this book has also benefited greatly from discussions with a number of people over the years: the students in my classes "AIDS to Writing" and "AIDS in the United States," the members of ACT UP/New York and ACT UP/RI, Robert Lee, Joanne Melish, Richard Meckel, Elizabeth Francis, Therese Jones, and the participants in the "Performing AIDS" conference. Thanks also to the staff at the Lesbian Herstory Archives and to ACT UP/New York archivist Stephan Jost for assisting me in accessing archival materials related to ACT UP/New York, as well as to the library staff and reference librarians at Brown and Harvard Universities. I am also indebted to John De Cecco and the staff at The Haworth Press, who helped shepherd this project toward its final form. Last but not least, I want to thank Jeff Sposato, who provided love, support, and a critical eye in many ways. Although not all of the people mentioned here will agree with my conclusions, I am grateful for the assistance each provided.

Sections of Chapters 1 and 2 of this book previously appeared in the article "'All They Needed': AIDS, Consumption, and the Politics of Class," published in the *Journal of the History of Sexuality* 8 (July 1997); a shorter version of Chapter 3 is scheduled to appear in the *Journal of Medical Humanities* 19 (Summer/Fall 1998), a special issue devoted to the "Performing AIDS" conference, where the ideas in the chapter were first presented. I am grateful to all parties involved for their permission to reprint this material.

Introduction

In March of 1997, the New York chapter of the AIDS Coalition to Unleash Power (ACT UP) celebrated its tenth anniversary. There was definitely much to celebrate: ACT UP had been responsible during its ten-year history for producing some of the most important advances in AIDS research and some of the most crucial improvements in the lives of people with AIDS, and a number of chapters (including the flagship one in New York) were still doing activist work in 1997. At the same time, there was much to mourn: the lives of activists lost to AIDS; the lack of energy and membership in ACT UP in comparison to its heyday in the late 1980s and early 1990s; and the fact that many of the battles that had been fought in 1987—such as price gouging for AIDS drugs—still needed to be fought in 1997 (ACT UP/New York would demonstrate on Wall Street on March 24, 1997, exactly ten years to the day of its first demonstration, which had also targeted Wall Street and the overpricing of drugs).[1]

In 1990, I became actively involved with the ACT UP chapter in Providence, Rhode Island, where I was a graduate student. As Chapters 1 and 4 of this book explain in detail, I found ACT UP/RI to be a vibrant activist base, a source of friendship and emotional support, and an organization laden with contradictions. From what I had read about the much larger ACT UP chapter in New York, it too seemed to be grappling with its own set of contradictions. While in ACT UP, I also began reading novels and watching plays about AIDS in order to help me make sense of my activist work, a project that proved fraught with complications as well. Eventually, I was able to organize my confusion about ACT UP, AIDS politics, and the literary response to AIDS into three questions:

1. *Why do people think ACT UP is such a "radical" organization?*

My first question stemmed from my impatience with ACT UP's "radical" reputation, which I felt bore little resemblance to the actual

1

workings of the group. To a certain extent, I *wanted* the Ivy League–educated men who made up the majority of ACT UP/RI during the early 1990s to put aside the coat-and-tie politics that we all seemed most comfortable with and start doing something "radical" (since after all, what was ACT UP if it wasn't "radical"?). But at the same time, I also wished that if other gay men and lesbians in Rhode Island realized how far from "radical" those of us in ACT UP really were, they might like us better as a group and as individuals.

2. *Why do ACT UP/RI members seem to spend more time socializing with each other than doing activism?*

I began posing this question to other members of ACT UP at the point in the group's history when more people were attending the social gatherings after ACT UP meetings than were attending the meetings themselves. Those at the meetings would call others who hadn't been in attendance and tell them where we were going out to dinner so they could join us, and frequently after dinner, people would go out dancing together. For a number of members whose sole involvement with ACT UP was to attend the ninety-minute weekly meetings, the number of hours they spent socializing with ACT UP members in a given week would often exceed the amount of time they contributed to working with the organization to improve the lives of people with AIDS and HIV. At the time, I found this preference both baffling and infuriating.

3. *Why does the imaginative literature about the AIDS epidemic get so bogged down in love stories?*

My concern with the literature of the epidemic also stemmed from what I thought were distractions from the work of a viable AIDS politics. As an AIDS activist who frequently found himself without a boyfriend, I'd had difficulty finding affirmation for my own political work within a literary response to AIDS in which the search for a lover had often assumed an importance equal to or greater than the struggle for a cure. Often, even reading or viewing those novels and plays sympathetic to and explicitly focused on activist struggle around AIDS made me want to spend more time in bars and clubs and less at demonstrations. How, I wondered, was a body of literature that could produce such a response supposed to be doing anything to help end AIDS?

This book was fueled, then, by dual motivations: a need to answer these questions for myself and a simultaneous need to engage in a major research project as part of my graduate program. As such, what follows constitutes something of a literary hybrid—activist document combined with scholarly investigation. The activist part of this investigation has kept me honest; I had been in ACT UP for quite a while before I decided to study it, and my commitment to the group overshadowed (some might say excessively) the investigation I would undertake. Since I felt I was honestly engaged with AIDS and ACT UP on the activist level, however, I felt entitled to engage with it as a scholarly problem. At the same time, the training I had had as a graduate student at Brown allowed me to ask questions of ACT UP that I felt hadn't been adequately asked—questions about where ACT UP's reputation came from, about money and class, and about the politics of literary representation.

Love and Anger takes as its subject the question of politics and political struggle, particularly as they relate to AIDS and ACT UP. In Chapters 1 and 4, I look closely at that organization. ACT UP chapters exist nationwide, but I have focused on only two for the purposes of this study: ACT UP/New York and ACT UP/RI. As I have already suggested, ACT UP/New York represents a logical choice for any investigation of the organization. Founded in 1987, ACT UP/New York was originally *the* ACT UP—the first chapter, and historically the largest. Despite the eventual appearance of ACT UP chapters around the country, ACT UP/New York continued to provide leadership for the movement, especially in areas of national concern such as work concerning experimental drugs. Likewise, ACT UP/New York organized many of the demonstrations associated with the group as a whole (most notably, the 1989 "Stop the Church" action at St. Patrick's Cathedral), and more often than not, it had its hand in important demonstrations that occurred outside of New York or that were organized by other ACT UP chapters.

But although ACT UP/New York (and, less often, ACT UP/San Francisco and Los Angeles) received most of the media attention, I was acutely aware as a member of a smaller ACT UP chapter that what New York activists did was only the tip of the iceberg in the ACT UP story. Moreover, the questions about ACT UP that troubled me so much had stemmed from my involvement in ACT UP/RI, not

ACT UP/New York. As such, I decided to do an additional analysis of my own ACT UP chapter as a comparative to ACT UP/New York, as well as to control against inaccurate generalizations based on the experiences of just one chapter. Since I was already a member of ACT UP/RI, a study of that chapter was particularly convenient. But I also felt that Rhode Island, a small state whose entire population is the same as the island of Manhattan, and a place lacking the pull that large cities have on gays and lesbians, would provide a good contrast with a gay mecca such as New York. If I could tease out similarities between the two chapters, I figured, I might be able to make some generalizations about the organization as a whole. Although this has certainly been the case, differences between the two chapters have proven instructive as well.

Although a good deal of my analysis in Chapter 1 is based on books and articles about ACT UP (especially histories, news coverage, and activist writings about particular demonstrations), what was available about ACT UP in the public domain was not always useful in addressing my concerns. I was interested in a relatively unseen side of ACT UP, one which belied the image of radicalism and militantism that had been peddled by media coverage and activist rhetoric alike. As such, I have based much of my discussion of ACT UP on participant-observation work I did with the group—both as an active member of ACT UP/RI from 1990-1993, and as a visitor to ACT UP/New York during the summer of 1993[2]—and I quote heavily in Chapters 1 and 4 from the interviews that I conducted with approximately thirty activists. Such a heavy reliance on activists' own words might strike some readers as excessively subjective, but such a degree of subjectivity was exactly what I was looking for, as a reprieve from "objective" sources that seemed to have little sense of what was really going on within the organization. At the same time, I have relied upon written sources, my own observations, and the opinions of the dozens of activists I spoke to (on tape and informally) in order to control against misleading comments from particular narrators.[3]

Chapters 2 and 3 consider four novels and plays written by a gay man or a lesbian with an involvement in ACT UP, each of which is concerned on the level of content with some kind of political response to AIDS.[4] Paul Monette's novel *Afterlife* contains a subplot about an AIDS terrorist who seeks revenge on a society that has turned its back on people with AIDS. Politics is also central to Larry Kramer's *The Normal Heart,* a semiautobiographical play that recounts the attempts of the Gay Men's Health Crisis to pressure the city of New York into responding to the growing epidemic. Two of the major characters in Tony Kushner's *Angels in America* are henchmen in the ongoing Reagan Revolution: the historical figure of Roy Cohn and a law clerk who writes reactionary decisions for an incapacitated federal judge. Sarah Schulman's novel *People in Trouble* tells the story of "Justice," an organization closely modeled after ACT UP/New York.

Chapters 1 and 2 of this study investigate the same problem—the way in which AIDS affected middle-class gay men *as a class.* In Chapter 1, I look at this problem in relation to ACT UP, and in Chapter 2, in relation to Monette's and Schulman's novels and Kramer's play. As such, Chapters 1 and 2 are preceded by an introduction that outlines the questions linking them, and the two chapters and the introduction to them are best read as a unit. Chapters 3 and 4 are connected as well, focusing as they both do on the intersection of erotic love and activist politics. If there is one central idea that unites my discussion of literature and activism in this book, it is that AIDS is a subject that binds eros and politics—a highly politicized disease whose agent (HIV) is frequently transmitted through sex, and which has disproportionately affected a community (gays) organized around its sexuality. Both Chapters 3 and 4 read fairly successfully on their own, although readers may find the context provided in Chapter 1 useful when reading about ACT UP in Chapter 4.

As of 1997 (when I write), ACT UP chapters still exist in many U.S. cities (including New York), and the imaginative response to the AIDS epidemic continues as strong as ever. Therefore, two choices I have made in this book need to be accounted for: my decision to stop my inquiry in 1993 and my decision to refer to ACT UP's work in the past tense. 1993 can be understood as a pivotal year—a sort of dramatic climax—for both AIDS activism and AIDS literature. 1993 was the year that Tony Kushner's epic *Angels in America* opened on Broadway, garnering a Pulitzer Prize, two Tony Awards for best play, and an unprecedented amount of national recognition in the process. No piece of AIDS literature had ever received as much mainstream attention before, and none (except perhaps for the musical, *Rent*) has received as much since. In terms of chronology, the New York production of *Angels in America* is the last imaginative text I consider, making 1993 a logical place to stop an inquiry into the literary response to AIDS.

1993 was an important year for ACT UP as well. As Chapter 1 of my book details, it was the year in which ACT UP/New York released its own version of a "Manhattan Project" for AIDS—the Barbara McClintock Project to Cure AIDS (later renamed the AIDS Cure Project). In doing so, ACT UP/New York brought down the curtain on the largely reformist agenda that had dominated the group during its first five years, so that 1993 represents something of the tail end of the version of ACT UP that I describe in this book. Moreover, as many commentators have noted, ACT UP had been undergoing a serious decline—in terms of money, energy, and membership—since about 1991, and I had a strong sense while doing fieldwork with ACT UP/New York that I was (regrettably) witnessing the beginning of the end of both the chapter and the movement. Although ACT UP/New York continued (and continues) to do important work (ACT UP/RI folded in 1995), conversations that I have had with ACT UP/New York members have served to confirm my suspicion. In referring to ACT UP in the past tense in this book, then, I do not wish to discount the work that many ACT UP chapters continue to do, but rather to recognize the fact that the ACT UP movement described in this study is very different from the one that exists today.

As all three of the questions that shaped this project should suggest, as much as this book has been a scholarly inquiry, it has also represented a personal voyage. Having attempted to answer these questions for myself, I hope I have come up with information that might prove useful for others who continue to work in the fight against AIDS.

PART ONE:
AIDS, GAY CULTURE,
AND THE POLITICS OF CLASS

Introduction to Part One

It is at the point where consumption converts its meaning
from a disease into a cure that we may begin to speak of a
consumer culture in the sense we experience it.[1]

—Jean-Christophe Agnew

For middle- and upper-middle-class gay men in the United States,
AIDS has constituted two kinds of crises: most obviously a health
crisis, but simultaneously a crisis of consumption. Accustomed to
having market access to whatever commodities they wanted, middle-
class gay men found themselves faced with an epidemic for which no
cure could be purchased because none existed.[2] As these men organized responses to their experience(s) of the epidemic, their efforts
were largely structured by a fundamental contradiction: their possession of a tremendous amount of class privilege, combined with their
inability to fully mobilize this privilege in the absence of a cure.

For men such as these, AIDS came as a rude shock, what I will refer
to in the following two chapters as a "class dislocation." This dislocation occurred along two lines. First, AIDS limited the ability of certain
gay men to pass as straight in the public sphere. Having been socialized into middle-class, heterosexual, (usually) white families, many of
these men had proven quite adept at juggling two identities before
AIDS: a private gay identity on the one hand, and a normative (i.e.,
heterosexual) public identity on the other. AIDS, in essence, outed
these men, marking them physically with the signs of a "gay disease"
and thereby fundamentally distancing them from the heterosexual
counterparts whose power, privilege, and material well-being they had
strived to attain.[3]

Second, AIDS dislodged certain gay men from their tenuous positions within the dominant classes by transforming unmarked *individuals* into members of a stigmatized *group*. The ability of gay men to

experience the privileges of straight men is dependent upon their ability to function socially as individuals. When gay men come together or are viewed as an identifiable group, they face discrimination and oppression; when they act alone, they can experience the privileges of most men. (Although there are few gay law firms, there are plenty of gay lawyers.) What AIDS represented was a *group* catastrophe: gay men (among others) were forced to appeal to the government and the public for needed assistance as a group, and they were in turn denied this assistance because of their membership in a group that the public deemed unworthy of concern.

Part One of this book examines two very different sites where the crises of class and consumption that I have just described were addressed: the AIDS Coalition to Unleash Power (ACT UP) and three pieces of imaginative literature—Paul Monette's novel *Afterlife,* Sarah Schulman's novel *People in Trouble,* and Larry Kramer's play *The Normal Heart.* My choice of such disparate examples is deliberate, since I believe that an interdisciplinary approach is crucial to an accurate understanding of cultural practice. In particular, my linkage of these very different examples represents a response to a tendency among practitioners of lesbian and gay studies to limit their attention to the study of texts. Although literary scholarship has taken a sharp turn toward the study of culture, the tendency of this scholarship to explain social and cultural phenomena primarily through readings of literary and visual texts has worked to narrow unnecessarily our understandings of broad cultural practices. Meanwhile, lesbian and gay studies has become a field dominated by scholars of literature, largely because of the acceptance and nurturance that English and literature departments have offered to the field.[4] As scholars in more empirically oriented fields such as history and anthropology have begun to note, however, such a disciplinary focus has meant that lesbian and gay studies practitioners have tended to shy away from empirical approaches in favor of a similarly narrow study of texts, with profound consequences for the field as a whole.[5] By contrast, the following chapters examine both a political movement and imaginative writings and, in doing so, attempt to suggest some of the ways in which anxieties over shifts in class and consumption structured a broad range of cultural practices by a generation of gay men devastated by AIDS—as well as some of the critiques that arose in response to these practices.

AIDS did not occur in a historical vacuum; nor did the processes described in the following chapters simply drop from the sky. Although the story I am about to tell focuses primarily on AIDS, what the class logic structuring these responses to the epidemic points to in the broadest sense is a profound and defining ambivalence within post-Stonewall gay culture—an ambivalence that has been particularly apparent among white, middle-class gay men. As my analysis will suggest, gay identity and culture are fraught with a number of contradictions and divisions that make gay men unique among "minority" and subordinate cultures: Gay men can pass as straight, either all the time or in selective contexts; gay men are born into a variety of socioeconomic backgrounds; many gay men do not come to identify as gay until well into adult life; many gay men identify as gay but do not partake of gay culture or community. What these divisions and contradictions have meant, then, is that many gay men have historically stood both inside and outside of dominant culture simultaneously.[6] For some gay men, their "outside" positioning has been the impetus for an engagement with activist politics. For others, however, their "inside" positioning has provided an opposing incentive to integrate and "pass"—to deny in their actions and their lifestyles the ways in which they are excluded from dominant culture.

As we shall see, by lumping gay men into an outcast group and forcing them to adopt the political tactics of the oppressed, AIDS constituted a moment in which the positioning of middle-class gay men in relation to dominant culture moved significantly toward the outside. If many gay men were ambivalent about their dual positioning before AIDS, however, the class dislocations that resulted from the epidemic only served to exacerbate these feelings. In fact, a number of the responses to AIDS created by these men have been premised on one of two notions: that they continue to remain "inside" dominant culture despite the epidemic, or that such a positioning is worth recovering. What makes a group such as ACT UP or a novel such as *Afterlife* particularly interesting, in fact, are the sparks produced when the ambivalence that many middle-class gay men already had about their positioning on the "outside" rubbed against a health emergency that demanded an oppositional practice, e.g., activism.

Although the following chapters can certainly be read as a critique of class privilege within segments of gay male culture, it is important to keep in mind that middle-class gay men suffer from multiple types of oppression within our society, including gay bashing and antigay discrimination. My argument in the following two chapters is not intended to trivialize this level of oppression. For one thing, although I will be focusing almost exclusively on class in my analysis, I do not wish to imply that class is the only important axis of identity in the lives of middle-class gay men (an assertion that would position such men as privileged but not simultaneously oppressed). Rather, my primary focus on class is simply intended to suggest that, in the absence of an AIDS cure, middle-class status could no longer function as the position of privilege that it used to be for many gay men.

Nor is the following argument intended to minimize the amount of suffering that white gay men and the white gay male community have undergone because of AIDS. Eric Rofes among others has done an excellent job of recounting the physical and psychological toll—the amount of death and suffering—that AIDS has produced within the white gay male community.[7] Readers should recognize, however, that to acknowledge the class privileges that structured both a movement such as ACT UP and the writings of certain of its members is not simultaneously to denigrate that movement or to cast aspersions on its participants (who, in fact, included myself). Nor is it to imply that the class privileges that many financially secure gay men have experienced in their lives have managed to wipe out their personal experiences with oppression. White, middle-class gay men have experienced quite enough death in the past fifteen years to render such a claim ridiculous.

It is also important to differentiate the argument that follows from a potentially homophobic discourse that positions gay men as frivolous overachievers in a consumer society. Barren of children, this argument goes, gay men have found themselves swamped with disposable income and have accordingly participated in an irresponsible consumption frenzy unavailable to heterosexuals. Gay and lesbian critics of this position have pointed out that gay men as a whole are not wealthier than their straight counterparts (and may in fact be slightly poorer), that such thinking is derived from media perceptions of gay men that ignore working-class gays (who tend to be less visible), and that gay disposable income can be easily eaten up in the caretaking of elderly parents or, increasingly, children.[8] Although this is certainly true, it is also true that men as a group still make considerably more money than women do in this country, so that a gay male couple with two male wage earners will, on average, have more income than a heterosexual couple with one male and one female wage earner—regardless of whether dependents are involved.[9]

Rather than taking sides in this debate, my own analysis looks at AIDS from another perspective—one which emphasizes class over sexuality. My description of AIDS as a "crisis of consumption" for middle-class gay men might at first glance appear to link homosexuality with consumption, but this is not my intention. Rather, the following two chapters view AIDS as a crisis of consumption for these men not because they are gay, but because they are middle class. Since AIDS has not widely affected middle-class heterosexual men in the United States, however, the crisis of consumption that I examine in these chapters is located primarily (although one could argue not strictly) within the gay male community.

This is not to say, however, that gay men have not developed a particularly problematic relationship to processes of consumption in ways besides their purported stockpiling of disposable income. In fact, the argument that follows intersects with a number of recent investigations into the role of consumption within gay culture. Anthony Freitas, Susan Kaiser, and Tania Hammidi have argued, for instance, that gay political subjectivity in the United States has become increasingly tied to the corporate recognition of gays as a target market, a particularly important signifier of "citizenship" in a consumer society.[10] Likewise, Nicola Field has criticized the extent to which particular commodities have been positioned as "common references" through which gay culture is understood to recognize itself—e.g., items targeted specifically to gay consumers (magazines, freedom rings) or the organization of mass-marketed commodities (furniture, clothing) into what is sometimes called gay style.[11] Although the following two chapters do not interrogate these positions directly, these arguments do raise some important questions. If consumption is constitutive of contemporary (middle-class) gay identity, we might ask, then what are the implications for gay subjects when consumption as a process becomes impossible? What happens to gay male culture when the one thing many gay men need to buy the most—a cure—is not for sale? And what kinds of responses—political and cultural—have developed in light of the class dislocation that has occurred as a result? In order to consider these and other questions, I turn my attention first to ACT UP.

Chapter 1

Acting Up:
AIDS and the Politics of Class

To go into a Catholic mass, in a beautiful cathedral in New York . . . and start throwing condoms around in the mass, I'm sorry, I think it sets back the cause. We cannot move to the extreme.[1]

—President George Bush, 1992

ACT UP/New York was founded in March of 1987, and Larry Kramer is generally given the credit—if not for creating the anger and energy that would fuel the organization, then for giving the speech at the Lesbian and Gay Community Center in New York that caused the anger and energy to crystallize.[2] ACT UP was created in the context of a burgeoning epidemic that showed no signs of ending, of a federal government whose response to the epidemic had been minimal at best, and of AIDS service organizations (such as the Gay Men's Health Crisis in New York) that, according to critics such as Kramer, had devoted most of their energies to service provision at the expense of political activism. Kramer's speech called for an AIDS organization that would be "devoted solely to political action," and his words struck a chord within a community in which certain segments had already begun to turn toward such a response.[3]

ACT UP/New York would always be the most celebrated, and arguably, the most important ACT UP, but almost eighty ACT UP chapters existed by 1993. Strictly speaking, all ACT UP chapters are spin-offs of ACT UP/New York, but ACT UP/New York's role in the genesis of the Rhode Island chapter was particularly direct.

On leave from college in 1987 and living in New York, Brown University student Stephen Gendin had agreed to attend Larry Kramer's March 10 speech in exchange for Kramer's participation in a conference that he was organizing. Gendin became a founding member of ACT UP/New York, an experience that he would bring back with him when he returned to Rhode Island in the fall of 1987, and he was one of six people arrested at ACT UP/RI's first major demonstration in May 1988.

ACT UP/New York's initial focus was quite simple: drugs. The cure was out there somewhere, and homophobic politicians, profit-obsessed pharmaceutical companies, and an antiquated federal bureaucracy were preventing it from reaching the people who needed it. The first ACT UP demonstration took place on March 24, 1987 on Wall Street; the focus was the unholy relationship between the Food and Drug Administration (FDA) and drug companies working on AIDS, especially Burroughs Wellcome, which had just announced a $10,000 per year price tag for its newly approved AIDS drug AZT. ACT UP gained nationwide notice within the gay community following its participation in the March on Washington for Lesbian and Gay Rights in October 1987, and by the time ACT UP/RI was founded in the spring of 1988, ACT UP had begun to expand its purview to include issues that were less directly relevant to the needs of its primarily middle-class, male membership. Although ACT UP/New York would continue its intensive and nationally respected research on drugs, pharmaceutical companies, and the federal AIDS bureaucracy through its Treatment and Data committee (T and D), dozens of other committees and caucuses formed over the next several years to address a diverse array of local, state, and national issues: women's lack of access to government-sponsored clinical trials, the treatment of homeless people with AIDS (PWAs), the workings of the insurance industry, the unavailability of condoms in New York public schools. Public attention, meanwhile, was focused on ACT UP's major demonstrations: at the FDA in 1988, the Fifth International Conference on AIDS in Montreal in 1989, the National Institutes of Health (NIH) in 1990, the Centers for Disease Control (CDC) in 1990, and perhaps most famously, St. Patrick's Cathedral in New York in 1989.

In the history of social and political movements in the United States, ACT UP is something of a standout, an anomaly during a decade in which the vibrant activism of the 1960s and early 1970s (second-wave feminism, black civil rights, the New Left) had largely been abandoned.[4] At the same time, ACT UP must also be understood as a something of a paradox—a movement for social change that was created in large part by individuals with a significant investment in the status quo. In ACT UP/New York and ACT UP chapters throughout the country, the majority of activists were white men, many of whom were quite well-off financially, and most of whom had little (if any) previous interest in or experience with grassroots activism.[5]

Professional, affluent, and unfamiliar with activist politics, these men came to ACT UP with a number of expectations and understandings: that dominant institutions (a capitalist economy, a pluralist political system) could and should work for them, that power was connected to institutional access and to whom one knew, that people would be willing to listen to what they had to say. Moreover, as white middle-class men, these activists came to ACT UP with a foothold in the dominant classes—a shaky foothold in light of AIDS, no doubt, but one that might be recoverable were the epidemic to somehow go away (which was, in the end, the goal of ACT UP). For many of its male members, in other words, ACT UP represented a political response not to fundamental social inequalities, but to the fact that their class position could not benefit them in the absence of a cure.

Not all ACT UP members were white, not all were gay, not all were men, and not all were financially secure. More important, not all gay white men in that organization possessed the same politics (as activists repeatedly reminded me, there were women and men, people of color and white people, etc., on both sides of every issue).[6] Nonetheless, two facts hold. First, *most* of the white men in ACT UP (as well as some women and people of color) came to that organization with certain understandings and experiences having to do with their class backgrounds—understandings that structured both their level of faith in existing institutions and the ways in which they were used to going about creating change.[7] Second, *all* white, middle-class gay men in ACT UP possessed a relationship to the dominant classes that women or people of color lacked—they could pass in certain contexts as white straight men and benefit socially and economically from doing so. This would occur regardless of politics: certain gay white men in ACT UP might be sincerely concerned about how AIDS affected women, poor people, and people of color, but it would always affect *them* differently. As a group, of course, white gay men are oppressed, as the AIDS epidemic has made painfully clear. But as individuals, white, middle-class gay men possess a relationship to the dominant classes that is defining, beneficial, and ultimately inescapable—whether in the workplace or in activist organizations.

In this chapter, I focus on the political consequences for ACT UP of what I will refer to as the "class style" of the majority of its members. I use the term "class style," rather than "class status" or "class background," because although almost everyone in ACT UP (male and female, white and nonwhite) was professional and middle class, only certain people in the group *acted* as though this entitled them to particular rights and privileges. This sense of entitlement was brought by these activists to the group and was translated into particular political assumptions and approaches: that existing institutions would come through for them, that getting access to powerful people was the best way to create change. Because their middle-class identities had appeared unmarked (at least before AIDS), white, middle-class gay men—whatever their professed politics—had been more able to operate under these assumptions than had women or people of color. Upon entering ACT UP, then, these men proved more likely to adopt such a class style than did others in the group.[8] Meanwhile, as we shall see, many lesbians in ACT UP had a background in feminist and other progressive politics that persuaded them that, whatever their own class backgrounds, existing institutions would never work for them in the same way that they would work for men. Nonetheless, since the majority of ACT UP members were white middle-class men, the class style of these men ultimately became the dominant style of the group as a whole, with pockets of dissent attempting to push it in other ways.

My argument in this chapter proceeds as follows. I begin by discussing ACT UP's reputation as a "radical" organization and explain where that reputation came from. I then consider the two main consequences of ACT UP's class makeup: its underlying commitment to the reform of existing institutions (which I discuss under "Goals") and the tendency of certain members to equate institutional access with the ability to create change (discussed under "Tactics"). In each of these two cases, I consider the ways in which the political approaches that resulted from these politics created for ACT UP important victories, as well as profound defeats that would ultimately cause ACT UP to reevaluate a number of its core beliefs.

REPUTATION

In the minds of most popular and scholarly commentators, ACT UP represented the vanguard of a new, radical gay movement. Fascinated by ACT UP's massive, colorful, and elaborately orchestrated demonstrations, by its use of symbols, and by its insertion of identity politics into its actions, these commentators viewed (and continue to view) ACT UP as subversive, destabilizing, threatening, and even revolutionary in nature. Although some of these assertions demonstrate a considerable level of confusion (such as a tendency to conflate "militant" demonstrations with "radical" agendas), others have represented useful ways of understanding at least some components of ACT UP's work. Although the majority of this chapter will focus on the ways in which ACT UP's actual workings belied its reputation, I want to begin here by mapping out what ACT UP's reputation was and then offering explanations for why it developed.

Since few people had actual firsthand exposure to an ACT UP demonstration, popular media accounts of ACT UP's street activism were crucial to the development of the group's reputation.[9] News coverage of ACT UP demonstrations, editorials and opinion pieces commenting on (and usually denouncing) ACT UP, and feature articles in a number of magazines presented readers with a picture of ACT UP as an angry, militant—and therefore dangerous—organization. Many journalistic accounts of ACT UP contained titles that were highly provocative in themselves, such as "Advocates' Tactics on AIDS Issues Provoking Warnings of a Backlash" *(The New York Times)*, "ACT UP Making Headlines—and Enemies" *(The Record)*, "The West Coast Gay Tantrum" *(New York City Tribune)*, and "Civil Disobedience vs. Uncivilized Behavior" *(New York Daily News).*[10] However, other pieces went on to criticize ACT UP at much greater length.

Shortly after ACT UP's 1989 demonstration at St. Patrick's Cathedral, for instance, the conservative pundit John Leo devoted his regular column in *U.S. News and World Report* to ACT UP. Titled "When Activism Becomes Gangsterism," Leo's column described ACT UP as "the No. 1 loose cannon of local politics, now powerful and feared," suggested that journalists were secretly referring to the group as *brownshirts,* and concluded with a warning to readers. "Support for the dignity and freedom of gays does not automatically mean overlooking the threat to our freedom by gangster groups such as ACT UP," Leo wrote.[11]

Leo also suggested that ACT UP had intimidated critics into keeping silent, as did Ray Kerrison, a columnist for the *New York Post.* Describing December 10, 1989, the day of "Stop the Church," as "the day that homosexuals unleashed their mad rampage through St. Patrick's Cathedral, defiling everything that is holy and sacred in the Catholic Church," Kerrison went on to complain that gay activists had entirely silenced their opponents "while reserving for themselves the right to use any defamation, insult, outrage, ridicule, or mockery."[12]

Even more sympathetic pieces could border on the sensationalistic. In March 1989, for instance, *The Washington Post* ran an overview of ACT UP's first two years with the inflammatory title, "Getting Militant about AIDS: Vandalism, Confrontations Mark Escalating Protest." In contrast to previous AIDS activism, the article noted in its third paragraph, ACT UP's version of AIDS activism now meant

> disrupting meetings to scream at public officials, pelting opponents with condoms, . . . leaving the chalked outlines of bodies on sidewalks and streets, plastering cities with "bloody" red hand-prints, employing the whole panoply of loud and sometimes illegal protest.[13]

The article was accompanied by four photos showing activists behaving in exactly this fashion, while descriptions of some of ACT UP's less dramatic doings (such as meeting with government officials) were buried deep within the piece.

Although heterosexual commentators were more likely to offer readers hyperbolic descriptions of ACT UP activities, a number of prominent gay commentators described ACT UP in a similarly alarmist fashion. In an article criticizing ACT UP's tactics at the 1989 International Conference on AIDS in Montreal, for instance, Randy Shilts argued that ACT UP's "methods are becoming so confrontational that they are beginning to backfire." "In the political arena," Shilts pointed out, "expressing anger for the sake of expressing anger is infantile, and sometimes counterproductive."[14] The popular gay philosopher Richard Mohr went even further than Shilts in his 1992 book *Gay Ideas*, describing as "acts of terrorism" ACT UP's protest at an exhibit of photographs of PWAs in New York, its "complete drowning out" of Health and Human Services Secretary Louis Sullivan at the 1990 International Conference on AIDS in San Francisco, and "Stop the Church."[15] Mohr was hardly a solitary voice in his criticism of "Stop the Church," either. Although gay and AIDS organizations throughout the country were generally supportive of the goals of the demonstration—such as calling attention to Cardinal John O'Connor's active opposition to gay rights, abortion rights, and condom use—most were critical of ACT UP's tactics inside the cathedral itself, including civil disobedience during O'Connor's sermon and one activist's crumbling of a communion host.[16] "Denouncing the spectacle inside St. Patrick's may take courage," one letter writer in *OutWeek* magazine noted, "but it is the only thing that can save the gay movement from its own lunatic fringe."[17]

Although journalists and other commentators were certainly justified in viewing ACT UP demonstrations as militant and outspoken (even as they tended to focus on these demonstrations over the rest of ACT UP's activities), these accounts contributed to an understanding of ACT UP as a "radical" organization as well. Such a move served to conflate tactics with goals, equating the outrageous tactics ACT UP used during demonstrations with what was presumed to be an equally outrageous social agenda. Although largely inaccurate (as we shall see shortly), conflations of ACT UP's tactics and goals are not all that surprising. As activists themselves suggested, in a political culture in which noninstitutional politics is largely unfamiliar, any kind of activism tends to be branded as extremist. "We're described as radical," Maxine Wolfe (NYC)[18] noted:

because what we do is not acceptable, polite lobbying. Because we do street actions, because we take over places, because we close down the FDA or lie down in St. Patrick's Cathedral, which are *claimed* not to be conventional American processes for political change. However, we did start with a revolution! . . . The ideology in the United States is that if you just went and you lobbied your congressperson, and they represent you, you would be fine. And so anything that's not like that is more radical.

Peter Hocking (RI) offered a similar opinion. "People in this country, even though it's allowable, just don't do that," he explained. "They don't spontaneously protest, and it's still something that people are really afraid of, especially when it's around identity politics, like sexual orientation, which AIDS in this country still is."

Popular commentators were not the only people to view ACT UP in this way, however. The rhetoric enlisted by ACT UP members and their supporters alike also contributed to understandings of ACT UP as a "radical" or even "revolutionary" organization. "Conditions are ripe for revolutionary behavior not when people feel oppressed, but when their rising expectations are dashed," ACT UP/New York member Bob Rafsky announced in a *Spin* Magazine article in 1989. "This community was born with high expectations: We were liberated, and the world was ours. Suddenly, we were dying, and nobody gave a shit. And those are conditions for revolution. It just took a while to sink in."[19] Contributing to ACT UP's reputation in this regard has been a line of thinking that has viewed ACT UP as the reviver of a derailed gay liberation movement committed to the overthrow of a social system predicated on sexist and heterosexist oppression.[20] Writing of ACT UP's work against homophobia, for instance, Douglas Crimp and Adam Rolston argued that "we see ourselves both as direct heirs to the early radical tradition of gay liberation and as rejuvenators of the gay movement, which has in the intervening decades become an assimilationist civil rights lobby."[21] Such a perception was echoed by the historian Martin Bauml Duberman at a ceremony commemorating the twentieth anniversary of the Stonewall Riots: addressing a crowd containing a large ACT UP contingent, Duberman suggested that the creation of ACT UP pointed to the beginnings of "a new gay movement which is once more radically oriented."[22]

As the pieces I have discussed so far should suggest, ACT UP's tactics played a pivotal role in the development of the group's reputation. Two components of these tactics in particular—ACT UP's civil disobedience and its "symbolic" activism—are worth considering in some detail, for they offer important clues as to why so many people viewed ACT UP as a "radical" organization. ACT UP's frequent and prominent use of civil disobedience was crucial to the development of media (and therefore popular) understandings of ACT UP as an irrational, unpredictable, or (to use the words of former President Bush) "extremist" organization, in large part because most of it was "indirect" in nature. As Carl Cohen has noted, civil disobedience usually assumes one of three forms: "direct civil disobedience," in which protesters violate the offending law itself (e.g., African Americans occupying seats at a segregated lunch counter); "indirect civil disobedience," in which the law violated is one only "symbolically" connected to the focus of the demonstration (e.g., blocking traffic to protest U.S. foreign policy); and "direct action," which Cohen describes as "unlawfully interfering with the allegedly immoral practice" (abortion clinic protesters violating trespassing laws in order to prevent women from getting abortions, not to demand an end to trespassing ordinances). Although the moral reasoning behind direct civil disobedience is usually readily apparent, practitioners of symbolic forms of civil disobedience have had a much more difficult time justifying their actions to outside observers.[23]

Although ACT UP's civil disobedience work occasionally fell within the category of "direct" civil disobedience (distributing clean needles as a means of protesting the illegality of such a practice, for instance), most of ACT UP's work in this area was indirect in nature, a fact that was not lost on commentators.[24] In a 1991 *San Francisco Chronicle* piece, for instance, Jon Carroll praised needle exchange efforts as being "in the best tradition of civil disobedience," but went on to criticize an ACT UP demonstration that involved blocking traffic on the Golden Gate Bridge. "Since when did Marin commuters have anything to do with anything?" Carroll asked. "In what way does making them uncomfortable . . . serve the goals of AIDS research or anti-discrimination?"[25] Certainly, any act of civil disobedience—no matter what form it takes—is likely to be viewed as extremist by some: even acts of direct civil disobedience that now appear to be of unquestionable justification were viewed by many as excessive at the time they were committed.[26] Nonetheless, given the frequently indirect nature of ACT UP's work in this area, combined with the fact, as Alvin Novick has noted, that ACT UP's civil disobedience is "*meant* to intrude, to provoke, to irritate, and to offend,"[27] civil disobedience contributed to an extremist reputation for ACT UP more readily than in the case of other movements.

Even more important than civil disobedience in the development of ACT UP's reputation, however, was ACT UP's deliberate manipulation of cultural codes—its symbolic activism—a component of ACT UP's repertoire that has attracted the attention of a number of academic commentators. Relying either explicitly or implicitly on recent understandings of movement politics made possible by theorists of the "new social movements," these commentators have located the impact of ACT UP outside of the traditional political realm of contests with the state, focusing instead on ACT UP's interventions in the area of "cultural" or "symbolic" politics. Unlike media overreactions to ACT UP's tactics, which demonstrate a rather limited understanding of ACT UP's work, these studies provide a useful way of understanding at least some of the impact ACT UP has had in this country.

As Joshua Gamson has concisely summarized, a number of European theorists have viewed "the movements of the 1960s and their apparent descendants—the peace movement, for example, or feminist, ecological, or local-autonomy movements . . . as 'new' phenomena to be accounted for; it is their nonrational focus on identity and expression that these theories emphasize as distinctive."[28] These theorists, notes Gamson, possess a "recognition that the field of operation has shifted, broadly put, to 'civil society' and away from the state; that culture has become more of a focal point of activity (through 'life-style' and 'identity' movements, for example)."[29]

Of all the writers on new social movements, Alberto Melucci has perhaps most closely mapped the types of "symbolic" activism associated with these groups. According to Melucci, symbolic forms of activism must be evaluated outside of a framework that privileges contests with the state. Although most commentators tend to "judge collective action in terms of its impact on the political system" (a move in line with traditional Leninist assessments of what constitutes political change),[30] Melucci focuses on what he calls the "pre-political and metapolitical qualities" of these movements. "Movements," he argues:

> operate in the pre-political dimensions of everyday life. Within its informal networks, collective actors collaborate in the laboratory work of inventing new meanings and testing them out. But movements also contain a metapolitical dimension. They publicize the existence of some basic dilemmas of complex societies which cannot be resolved by means of political decisions.[31]

Today's movements provide "symbolic challenges to the dominant codes";[32] they function both to "enlighten what every system doesn't say of itself, the amount of silence, violence, irrationality which is always hidden in dominant codes" and to "announce to society that something 'else' is possible."[33] As such, Melucci argues, new social movements possess "a conflictual and antagonistic, but not a political orientation, because they challenge the logic of complex systems on cultural grounds."[34]

As a number of commentators have noted, ACT UP's work (and especially its street activism) can also be understood in terms of the symbolic activism that Meluci and others have described. ACT UP's demonstrations, although ostensibly focused on traditional targets (bureaucrats, the president), were often only partially oriented toward the creation of legal or institutional reform. Although ACT UP trademark activities such as "kiss-ins," "die-ins," and "outing" frequently occurred within the context of demonstrations focused on traditional political demands, such as more AIDS research, these activities simultaneously functioned as a type of cultural activism that did its work outside of demands on the state.[35]

One writer who has done an extensive assessment of ACT UP's relationship to the new social movement paradigm is Joshua Gamson.[36] Gamson locates ACT UP's symbolic activism in the lesbian and gay identity of most ACT UP members. Although ACT UP demonstrations frequently focused on everyday targets such as the media, the "medical establishment," drug companies, and government agencies—a type of activism, Gamson argues, in which "AIDS politics and gay politics are quite separable"[37]—ACT UP also participated in a form of symbolic activism that addressed AIDS through interventions concerning homosexuality. In today's society, Gamson explains in a Foucauldian move, "power is maintained less through direct force or institutionalized oppression and more through the delineation of the 'normal' and the exclusion of the 'abnormal.'" As such, he argues, "activists use the labels to dispute the labels and use their abnormality and expressions of gay identity to challenge the process by which normality was and is defined."[38] Activists "take a symbol used to oppress [such as the pink triangle] and invert it," or engage in a form of "boundary-crossing" in which "ACT UP . . . seizes control of symbols that traditionally exclude gay people or render them invisible, and take them over . . . and *make them mean differently*."[39] In doing so, ACT UP managed to tackle on a symbolic level homophobia and AIDS-phobia simultaneously "at a time when the stigma of disease has been linked with the stigma of deviant sexuality."[40]

I cite these theorists at some length because they provide a useful means of understanding where so much of ACT UP's reputation came from and why this reputation was, in part, deserved. In a country in which "politics" is viewed as a national pastime but cultural change is considered a threat, ACT UP activities that made symbolic as well as institutional interventions represented one of the primary reasons why ACT UP was viewed by so many as a "radical" organization. For activists seeking to create changes within government and drug companies as quickly as possible, the symbolic work done by ACT UP demonstrations was often viewed as a distraction from the group's primary focus. For other activists with a less directed agenda, however, symbolic activism represented an important end in itself, challenging the heterosexist foundations of American society in a manner that should be measured not in terms of politicians swayed or reforms won, but in terms of the amount of horror, confusion, chaos, and disapproval such actions could produce.

Many ACT UP demonstrations were ready-made, in fact, for the occurrence of "secondary" symbolic effects. As the criticisms of ACT UP noted above may have already suggested, part of the actual attractiveness of ACT UP demonstrations for participants was their ability to provide an outlet for the expression of anger and grief resulting from homophobia and the ravages of AIDS, as well as to create a safe space for the display of a stigmatized sexuality that many would prefer to see kept under wraps. Critics such as Gamson are correct in suggesting that ACT UP members deliberately pushed sensitive cultural buttons at demonstrations—certainly with the intention of doing more than changing the minds of bureaucrats or drug company officials.[41] Given their generally undisciplined nature, in fact, ACT UP demonstrations practically invited unplanned activities by individual members—activities that could alter the tone of an entire demonstration, with no "opportunity" for the group as a whole to distance itself from the actions of more extremist members.[42]

Such "renegade" activism occurred frequently throughout the histories of both ACT UP/New York and ACT UP/RI and usually attracted a disproportionate share of media attention. For instance, despite the presence of 5,000 people at "Stop the Church," most of whom demonstrated peacefully outside the cathedral, the crumbling of a communion wafer by just one member came to represent the entire demonstration in the eyes of the media and the public. Likewise, during my summer of fieldwork with ACT UP/New York, a group of us participated in what was intended to be a silent informational zap at a reception for newly installed White House AIDS Coordinator Kristine Gebbie (a quickly organized and implemented demonstration or protest). ACT UP/New York members holding a banner on the stage in front of Gebbie stood helpless, however, while a handful of members of ACT UP/DC used the opportunity to shout Gebbie down, which, although not part of ACT UP/New York's original plan, was described as the purpose of the demonstration in subsequent media coverage.

ACT UP/RI had a similar experience in 1990, when media coverage of an otherwise restrained picket line outside of a Bill of Rights exhibit zeroed in on the actions of one participant, who burned an American flag and then entered the display and screamed at bystanders.[43] Affinity-group activity during demonstrations, although purportedly separate from official ACT UP tactics, also tended to have the effect of altering the tone of the demonstration approved by the group as a whole. This is not to suggest, however, that members usually found these occurrences unacceptable; in fact, the enthusiasm with which many activists greeted the unsanctioned activities of affinity groups or individual members is indicative of the extent to which ACT UP demonstrations—with the consent of many (although certainly not all) members—were understood as a space in which anything might potentially occur.

If ACT UP should *not* be understood as a "radical" organization, it is because the majority of its work was ultimately not focused on any kind of "root" solutions—a position that I will argue in greater detail in the remainder of this chapter. At the same time, such a reputation endured, and not without reason. Activists themselves realized that ACT UP attracted new members (and repelled potential allies) because of the image its tactics created, and that it achieved a sense of group identity through its reputation as much as its actions. Even if ACT UP never aimed for the overthrow of the American government (or even of the FDA, for that matter), ACT UP's symbolic politics achieved—and, in my opinion, were intended to achieve—a variety of effects that went beyond simply attracting reporters or pressuring bureaucrats in order to produce reforms. On at least one level, these tactics managed to annoy, frighten, and create an atmosphere of chaos, to disrupt normal cultural patterns, and to send a message to those watching on the street or in their homes that the lives of people who were not confronted by AIDS on a daily basis were not as safe as they might have thought. And if such a project was not in itself "radical," it certainly had very little to do with reform.

GOALS

ACT UP's symbolic activism is an important part of the story of that organization, and it was crucial to the development of popular understandings of the group. At the same time, these activities were not the only part of this story, nor, I want to argue, the most important. ACT UP's work (and especially its street activism) can productively be understood in terms of the new social movements, certainly, but ACT UP must be viewed as a political movement as well, one whose activities were ultimately geared to producing industry and (especially) state responses to the epidemic.

My definition of "politics" and the "political" here needs to be explained for it is considerably more traditional than some of the more expansive understandings of the "political" that have circulated in the past thirty years.[44] "Politics" and "political struggle" in this study are closely linked to the question of which public institutions have monopolies over mass resources, and it links capital and government accordingly. For the purpose of this discussion, I define "politics" as either (1) contests with the state or industry (e.g., AIDS activists versus the FDA, activists versus Burroughs Wellcome), (2) contests within the state (e.g., the President versus Congress, Senator Jones versus Senator Smith), or (3) contests between parties with competing agendas for the state (e.g., AIDS activists versus the religious right).[45] This definition is admittedly somewhat narrow; most noticeably, it fails to take into consideration the fundamental insight of the feminist movement that "the personal is political." I use this definition, however, because so much of ACT UP's work was premised on the notion that only the resources that the state and, to a lesser extent, industry could mobilize would be sufficient to end the epidemic. Volunteer organizations and charities could address certain needs of PWAs, but only the state had the ability to provide AIDS-related services at needed levels, and only drug companies or federally funded researchers had access to the kinds of financial resources necessary to develop and produce needed drugs. Thus, although many types of "political struggle" function independently of what government and industry will and will not do (focusing, for instance, on cultural interventions), ACT UP insisted that a "political" response to AIDS was inseparable from the workings of these public institutions.[46]

The Nature of Reform

When one views ACT UP in terms of its *political* effects, the picture I have already presented in this chapter begins to change dramatically. Although ACT UP's street activism may indeed have had destabilizing (even radical) cultural effects, ACT UP proved extremely unradical in a number of political areas, including an overall agenda that was primarily reformist in nature.

ACT UP's commitment to a reform politics occurred on two levels. First, despite the impression that may have been conveyed by the fervency of ACT UP's demonstrations, the organization's goals were always moderate in nature. Although a few ACT UP members promoted agendas focused on broad social changes such as the eradication of racism, sexism, and class inequalities, most members were primarily committed to the much narrower agenda of finding a cure for AIDS and ending the epidemic. Second, ACT UP displayed a continual willingness to use existing institutions to achieve those goals. Even as it attacked particular government agencies such as the FDA or the NIH or the price-setting policies of a particular pharmaceutical company, ACT UP's goal for much of its history was to reform the practices of such agencies and companies, rather than to eliminate them altogether. Although a "radical" politics might have been focused on "root" solutions such as the elimination of the FDA or the elimination of the capitalist approach to drug development, ACT UP operated for its first several years on the premise that rel-atively minor tinkering with existing institutions and practices could adequately address the needs of people with HIV.[47]

Several of ACT UP's most important projects—and greatest successes—were oriented along these lines. In 1988, for instance, ACT UP chapters from around the country joined forces in attacking the approval process that the Food and Drug Administration required for all new drugs entering the U.S. market.[48] The assault on the FDA represents the best example of ACT UP's initial faith in the idea that minor reforms brought about by activist pressure could produce a rapid end to AIDS: many ACT UP members were convinced that a cure for AIDS already existed but was languishing in the "drug pipeline," held up by a Byzantine drug-approval process that was entirely inappropri-ate for a fatal disease.[49] Given that, as one member put it at the time, "the FDA is using the same regulatory process with Tylenol as they are with AIDS drugs,"[50] ACT UP organized its demonstration around a number of demands: that the FDA "shorten the drug approval pro-cess," that it "ensure immediate free access to drugs proven safe and theoretically effective," and that it refuse to accept data from drug trials that employed the use of placebos (which would effectively keep some participants away from the drug they had entered the trial to access in the first place).[51]

The campaign against the FDA culminated in October 1988 with ACT UP's biggest national action to date—its "Seize the FDA" demonstration at FDA headquarters in Rockville, Maryland. One hundred seventy-six activists were arrested during the day-long dem-onstration, which managed to produce almost immediate changes in the way AIDS drugs were approved in the United States. Within a year of "Seize the FDA," four new AIDS drugs had received FDA licensing, and four other drugs had been made available through expanded access programs.[52] As activists soon discovered, no cure was waiting in the wings. However, changes in the FDA approval process did help to save or extend lives: drugs that slowed the progression of HIV or that prevented the development of opportunistic infections became available to people with AIDS much faster than they would have under previous FDA regulations.

Following the realization that the FDA's drug-approval process was not in fact preventing an existing cure from reaching the market, ACT UP turned its attention to the process of drug trials themselves. ACT UP's primary target in this regard was the AIDS Clinical Trials Group (ACTG), the series of federally sponsored drug trials conducted by the NIH. Here again, activists demonstrated a commitment to the idea that the creation of reforms in one agency (in this case the NIH) might be just the trick necessary to bring about a cure for either AIDS itself or for the numerous opportunistic infections that actually made people with AIDS sick.[53] As ACT UP viewed the situation, the ACTG was putting too many eggs in one basket, organizing the majority of its trials around nucleoside analogues such as AZT, a highly toxic drug that had already been approved by the FDA, and devoting little attention to either other classes of drugs or to treatments for opportunistic infections. In May 1990, over 1,000 activists from ACT UP chapters around the country descended on the NIH campus in Bethesda, Maryland, for ACT UP's "Storm the NIH" demonstration. Reciting a mantra of "Ten years. A billion dollars. One drug. Big deal." to call attention to the fact that the only drug that had been developed in the previous ten years for use against HIV was in fact AZT, activists brought national attention to the ways in which government scientists were mismanaging the federal fight against AIDS. ACT UP insisted that the NIH widen its investigations to include other kinds of drugs. At the same time, believing that access to trials currently being conducted might mean access to a potential, unreleased cure, activists also demanded that the NIH end the frequent practice of excluding women and people of color from government-sponsored drug trials. Because of the demonstration, immediate changes in the ACTG process did occur: for instance, activists were allowed to attend the Ninth ACTG meeting in June 1990 as official registrants for the first time.[54]

ACT UP's campaign to change the CDC definition of AIDS was a third ACT UP project based on the idea that small changes in existing institutions could have a major impact on the lives of people with HIV. The campaign against the CDC was premised on the idea that the CDC definition of AIDS had been developed around the opportunistic infections that had been experienced by a small group of gay men. Because of this, activists argued, women suffering solely from opportunistic infections such as pelvic inflammatory disease or cervical cancer—infections that were common in women but that were not included in the original definition—remained ineligible for an official AIDS diagnosis, depriving them of access to benefits and drug trials restricted to PWAs. Moreover, without guidelines directing health care providers to look for women-specific symptoms, many women with HIV would go undiagnosed until dangerously late. Joined by women from around the country, many with HIV, ACT UP members organized demonstrations at the CDC in January and December of 1990 after meetings with government officials failed to produce results. Following the demonstrations, ACT UP pressure against the CDC continued, and the CDC began a gradual process of amending its AIDS definition in August 1991.[55]

Closely tied to ACT UP's commitment to reform politics—to the idea that minor changes in existing institutions could adequately address the needs of PWAs—was ACT UP's insistence that only the resources that could be mobilized by the state would be adequate to address the magnitude of AIDS. Admittedly, such an insistence on the primacy of state power has been an important component of a number of radical movements, such as American socialism. But, in contrast to movements that have linked this insistence to the need to *replace* existing government institutions, for many years ACT UP acted almost exclusively on the premise that existing institutions would be adequate to the task of ending AIDS. As ACT UP/New York's Berna Lee noted, unlike political movements that have targeted specific institutions under the belief that "if you get rid of that institution, maybe things will get better . . . what we [ACT UP] want is for these institutions to do what we want them to do: we don't want to get rid of them." Government agencies might require reforming, and bureaucrats might need to have their minds changed on certain issues. Nonetheless, in contrast to radical movements in the history of this country, ACT UP was generally willing to work with the agencies and institutions already in place.[56]

Such a willingness applied to individuals as well. Contrary to the impression that ACT UP's relentless criticism of specific politicians and bureaucrats (such as former presidents Reagan and Bush or NIH scientist Anthony Fauci) could impart, ACT UP as a rule did not endorse individual candidates or politicians. Instead, it proved willing to work with any politician, bureaucrat, or industry official—of any party, and with any prior record—who was willing to support ACT UP's agenda. Committed to producing rapid change, ACT UP members turned immediately to those who already possessed power, rather than questioning whether this power was deserved; likewise, government and industry scientists with considerable knowledge about AIDS were viewed by ACT UP as potential partners—albeit partners who sometimes needed their minds changed. Larry Kramer for one was notorious for lauding government and industry players when they agreed to develop the projects of activists, but then castigating the same individuals when their agenda differed from that of ACT UP's (Kramer, for instance, labeled Fauci everything from a "murderer" to a "hero.").[57]

Such an accommodationist approach to AIDS activism was not inevitable. In fact, in a rather unorthodox reading of the history of the Gay Men's Health Crisis (GMHC), the first AIDS service organization in New York, Philip Kayal has argued that the early GMHC was a more "radical" organization than ACT UP, given its rejection of government involvement in the New York gay community's response to AIDS in favor of community-based response and empowerment. Deeming ACT UP's baseline claims on the state as "system-maintaining accommodation,"[58] Kayal understands GMHC as:

> the context within which the volunteer goes about creating an autonomous jurisdiction (a liberated zone) in which the work of nurturing and healing a dying people (the necessary work in AIDS) takes place. This is fundamentally political and radical because GMHC is holding together the fabric of life—human connections—for a whole endangered community and empowering it at the same time. (p. 91)

"Given the prevailing moral meaning of AIDS (and its deeper meaning for gays)," Kayal concludes, "to force an interior change of attitudes and feelings about the self and the community is the ultimate political statement, not angry street demonstrations directed at institutions."[59]

Kayal's argument here is obviously overstated: although community building certainly represents a particular kind of political work (see Chapter 4 of this book), Kayal fails to consider that any understanding of "healing" in the context of AIDS must involve not only spiritual healing via community formation, but also physical healing through treatments and ultimately a cure, something an AIDS service organization such as GMHC was less capable of working toward than an activist organization such as ACT UP. Moreover, Kayal himself is forced to admit by the end of his book the increasing role of government funding in GMHC's operations.

Nonetheless, Kayal's contrast between ACT UP and GMHC is a useful one, for it recognizes the extent to which ACT UP's project was grounded in the belief that a truly adequate response to AIDS would have to come from the state.[60] In contrast to GMHC, a service provider by nature, ACT UP generally viewed service provision as the government's work. Even in those rare instances when ACT UP *did* provide services, it did so only because government agencies had refused to or because the services being provided were illegal, and it always viewed its work on such projects as temporary.[61] When ACT UP/New York's Youth Education Life Line (YELL) distributed AIDS information and safer sex materials to New York City public school students, for instance, they did so only until they were able to convince city officials to institute a more comprehensive AIDS curriculum and to provide condoms in the schools.[62] And when needle activists in ACT UP/New York provided free, clean needles to injection drug users during a period when all needle possession in the city was illegal without a prescription, they conceived of their work both as civil disobedience and as a means of pressuring city and state officials to allow for legal needle exchanges, eventually forcing the issue into the courts.[63]

Not surprisingly, some members of ACT UP criticized such instances of service provision as "doing the government's work," a role they viewed as inconsistent with the mission of a direct action organization.[64] For the most part, however, such service provision was understood as a temporary measure that would end once outside agencies took over, optimally on a much larger scale than a group of part-time activists could ever provide. Once needle exchange became legal, for instance, ACT UP/New York dropped its sponsorship of such activity in favor of neighborhood organizations that were now at liberty to run the exchanges themselves, turning its activist attention to the unavailability of legal needles outside of the exchanges.

To a certain extent, ACT UP's commitment to the kind of reformist politics I have just described was linked to the fact that such a politics was the most expedient. With friends, lovers, and (in some cases) themselves sick or dying, most ACT UP members accepted the need to abandon a long-term politics focused on structural types of change in favor of more readily winnable battles having to do with treatments or a cure. "There are a lot of people in that room," Mary Cotter (NYC) explained:

> . . . that are, in and of themselves, true revolutionaries. . . . But I also think that, at the same time, there's so much death around us on a constant regular basis, that it stops us. . . . Because it's like, I'm concerned about today, and tomorrow, and my friends who are dying and continuing to die, and I want something done right here and right now. And so, I think it's really hard sometimes to kind of plan to smash the state, because that's a really long-term goal! [Cotter laughs] . . . whereas something like getting the HIV ban lifted and getting people released from Guantanamo Bay is real and tangible and happened.[65]

Such a degree of pragmatism, however, occasionally alienated individuals who came to ACT UP looking for a broader type of politics. "The problem with a lot of the new people who came into ACT UP," Stephen Gendin (NYC/RI) explained:

> was they were too radical. They wanted to end racism and end sexism and things like that, and they wanted a whole new, brighter world where everybody was healthy and happy. And dedicated treatment activists were like, "Let's increase the number of people taking this drug from one to ten, and we'll find ten people who are rich enough and wealthy enough to pay for

it, but it's better to have ten people taking it than one person taking it." And that's not a very radical concept. I mean, that's a very expeditious concept, and expediency I think was more than anything else the concept of ACT UP.

Equally as important to the development of ACT UP's commitment to reform as simple expediency, however, was the class background of the majority of its members. Cindy Patton has argued that gays felt entitled to make AIDS-related claims on the state because they were seen (or at least saw themselves) as a distinct minority group, but I would offer a competing explanation: at least as far as the men in ACT UP were concerned, claims on the state were based not on a sense of being members of a minority group, but rather on a sense of being members of the dominant classes.[66] As middle-class white men, many of whom had high-paying professional jobs, the majority of ACT UP members had no desire to radically alter government or to overthrow a capitalist system of production because existing institutions had always done well by them—extremely well, in some cases. Moreover, not only did these activists believe that a capitalist economy and a pluralist form of government had worked for them in the past and could work for them in the future (once the appropriate bugs had been worked out, of course), they also believed that such institutions *should* work for them—that they were entitled to have the state respond to their needs. Certainly, not everyone in ACT UP felt this way, but since decisions in both ACT UP/New York and ACT UP/RI were made on a majority vote basis, those who did feel this way were able to exert extensive influence on the workings of the group as a whole, even though women and people of color made up sizable minorities within the organization (especially in New York).[67]

Contrasting the markedly different attitudes about creating change (political and otherwise) that gay men and lesbians brought to ACT UP is an extremely useful way to see how much of ACT UP's agenda was defined—and ultimately circumscribed—by the class style of the majority of its members. Although far fewer women than men joined ACT UP/New York in the first place, those who did came to the organization with a much greater level of previous activist involvement than did the men. The women in ACT UP/New York, according to B.C. Craig (NYC), were primarily:

> lesbian feminists who had been at the forefront of many different kinds of activism for a long time, about pro-choice stuff and about antiwar stuff, lesbian and gay stuff, who had been active for a long time, and had a commitment to social change, an agenda about activism and a long-term commitment.

By contrast, many of the men who joined ACT UP—including a number of those who would come to assume leadership roles in the group—had no previous activist involvement but had been driven into an activist organization by either their own sickness or the sickness of a loved one.[68]

But if the men in ACT UP/New York had little political experience, what they did bring to that organization was a motivating sense of entitlement. Prior to coming to ACT UP, Craig explained, women activists had never imagined:

> that they were ever going to get anything. They just felt like they had to be a voice of dissension. I was one of them. We would stand outside and yell because somebody had to stand outside and yell. But it never occurred to us that anything was going to change, that anyone was going to listen to us, or that we would ever get inside.

By contrast, many of the men in ACT UP/New York came to that organization assuming that they were entitled to a response from the government and that they could force the government to produce such a response. Most of the men in ACT UP, according to Craig "couldn't believe that the system wasn't going to respond to them. And they had a sense of entitlement: 'I have a right to good medical care; you owe it to me! You have to give it to me, and you're lying, and I can know as much as you can. There's no reason that you're an expert and I'm not.'"

In part, such attitudes had to do with the fact that most of these men had no previous experience in grassroots organizing and had consequently never had to face the frequent reality checks about creating change that go hand in hand with progressive activism. At the same time, I would argue, these attitudes stemmed from the experience these men had had in the workday world: used to getting people to do what they wanted on a daily basis, many men came to ACT UP assuming that government and industry officials would eventually do their bidding as well. "As a majority white gay male group," Maxine Wolfe (NYC) explained:

> people weren't used to the world not changing for them. People would get out on the street and do some demonstration, and they'd expect the world to collapse. And when it didn't, they would get really upset. Because you know a lot of them ran offices where they said, "Get me coffee," and the coffee came; they said, "Make money," and the money was made.

The paradoxical context within which many ACT UP members operated was perhaps best summarized by Michelangelo Signorile in a 1989 interview in *Spin* magazine. "We're *from* the system," Signorile explained. "We're gay, but we are running companies, we are working for corporations, we are working for medical facilities, we are legal people. In a way, we're the same system that we're fighting."[69] Having benefited greatly from existing institutional arrangements earlier in their lives, many ACT UP members were reluctant to advocate (or even imagine) an agenda that would do anything besides make small changes in the ways that a handful of government agencies and pharmaceutical companies were dealing with AIDS. Likewise, many of the gay men in ACT UP approached activism with an ingrained belief that there was nothing fundamentally wrong with the way the U.S. government worked—that is, nothing that could not easily be fixed. As a survey conducted by Elbaz in 1989 indicated, for instance, men in ACT UP/New York "seem[ed] to believe in the official political system" much more than women did (although the tendency of women to vote actually decreased while they were in ACT UP, men continued to vote at high rates).[70]

This is not to deny that many ACT UP members (including some men) came to that organization with a more leftist or progressive politics. Nonetheless, these activists tended to bracket these politics in favor of the reform agenda that I have already described, primarily for two reasons. In the first place, as Craig explained, ACT UP/New York set out to avoid "becoming . . . a fringe group," one in which "lots of people affected by AIDS wouldn't feel like they were welcome."

Instead, as its name suggests, ACT UP imagined itself from the outset as being a "coalition," which meant that the politics of individuals with whom more radical members might disagree would have to be accommodated. Early in its history, in fact, ACT UP fought off attempts by both the International Socialist Organization and the New Alliance Party—two leftist organizations—to seize control of the group's agenda.[71]

ACT UP's agenda was organized around a "lowest common denominator" politics: in order to keep the group as large and diverse as possible, activists stuck closely to those projects that would be agreeable (or at least not offensive) to the vast majority of members, many of whom possessed moderate or even conservative politics. "I don't think that the majority of people in ACT UP are necessarily left-wing ideologues," Michael Swirsky (NYC) explained. "Many of them are people who want a cure. Certain ideas may be attractive to them: I know of very few right wingers in ACT UP. But occasionally you do find people who are conservative in political thought, but nonetheless share the goal of finding a cure." Sarah Schulman (NYC) echoed Swirsky's assessment, noting that ACT UP was a politically diverse group of people whose only commonality was either having AIDS or knowing someone who did, and whose pre-AIDS politics tended to change very little upon joining the organization. "There are people," Schulman noted:

> who were extremely radical and extremely analytical, and really willing to be transformed, and who had a broad view. . . . And, there have also always been people who were individualists, who did not really see other kinds of people as fully human, who desperately needed the approval of straight men. . . . People who were bond traders, and were just totally out for money, and totally apolitical . . . before they were infected or before their boyfriend was infected, and became activists, many of those people operated in ACT UP like they did on the floor of the stock exchange.

A second reason why activists with a more radical politics agreed to ACT UP's reformist agenda was because they too subscribed to the idea than an expedient approach was necessary in the context of a health emergency. Mary Cotter and Berna Lee were two ACT UP/

New York activists I spoke to who identified themselves as having a radical politics but who nonetheless felt comfortable working within ACT UP. For them, ACT UP represented a useful way to address one component of their larger political agenda—ending AIDS.

> **Cotter:** I'm not looking for an *AIDS* activist organization that's going to go smash the state; I'm looking for an organization that's going to smash the state on a bigger level [than just AIDS issues].

> **Lee:** If that type of a movement started, Mary and I would be creaming our pants.

> **Cotter:** Exactly. But that's not AIDS activism to me. . . . That's not what I look to ACT UP for. . . . When you're dealing with broad social issues, like sexism, racism, homophobia, I mean— reform versus revolution? It's like, come on! There's no question: of course it's revolution. You know, we've tried reform; it doesn't work. But, with something like AIDS: underneath all that, if the whole health care system were completely restructured, if homophobia didn't exist, if sexism didn't exist, if racism didn't exist, we would not be at this point in the crisis where we're at. Plain and simple. But we're here, right here and now, and because we can't reverse that, and because people are dying right now, this day, this minute, I want to do something right here and now that's going to end that now.

> **Lee:** And ACT UP is not the here all and end all for either of us, I don't think. Yes, if we ever do find a cure, lots of people are still going to be fucked, people of color are still going to be fucked, and women are still going to be fucked, and so are poor people. So, in that sense it's not radical enough. . . . But that's not what it's for.

As this exchange demonstrates, both Cotter and Lee felt that ACT UP was not—and was not intended to be—a forum in which they could work toward the broader social changes they both desired. Nonetheless, both women agreed that such work should be conducted in other organizations, and that ACT UP was to be valued instead for the work that it had proven itself capable of doing in the more limited context of the AIDS epidemic.

Because white middle-class men formed the majority of ACT UP, and because other activists were willing to accommodate their politics for the reasons I have just described, the class style of these men came to structure ACT UP in a fundamental way—so fundamental, in fact, that even when activists critiqued these biases, they did so in a way that was grounded in the notion that "the system" would eventually work for the men in the group. As Lee's final comment in the above quote might suggest, one of the earliest radical critiques to come out of ACT UP was that the emphasis that ACT UP had been putting on finding a cure (ACT UP's "drugs into bodies" agenda) might benefit people who could afford such a cure but would be useless for those who could not—primarily people of color and women in this country.[72] Such a perspective was intended as a critique of the short-sighted thinking that dominated the early years of ACT UP; at the same time, it was premised on the notion that ACT UP's reform agenda, however it might fail poor people in this country, would eventually work for those with enough money—that is, for the kinds of men who were drawn to ACT UP. With adequate reforms, the thinking went, government and industry would produce a cure—or at least useful treatments—and middle-class gay men would be able to afford them. Such a critique was generally launched by activists who were unsympathetic toward the class inequalities that exist in this country, and it was intended to motivate ACT UP to include in its agenda larger structural changes that would make treatments available to anyone who needed them. Nonetheless, this critique clearly demonstrates that even those in ACT UP who possessed a more radical politics were convinced that, given a little pushing, existing institutions would ultimately come to the rescue of middle-class gay men.

In terms of its membership demographics, ACT UP/RI was no exception to the pattern I have just established: most of its members during its seven-year history (and especially in its later years) were gay white men with professional jobs and Ivy League backgrounds, many of whom were more comfortable putting on coats and ties than demonstrating in the street. Nonetheless, ACT UP/RI's agenda, although also reformist in nature, was very different from that of ACT UP/New York, due in large part to the local political climate in Rhode Island.

Rather than attempting to get government *more* involved in addressing AIDS, as ACT UP/New York frequently did, ACT UP/RI was often more concerned with trying to prevent the Rhode Island state government from interfering in the lives of people with HIV. For instance, even as ACT UP/New York was focusing most of its energies on pressuring the federal government to produce a cure, ACT UP/RI tended to prioritize state infringements upon privacy, especially in the area of HIV and CD4+ (T-cell) testing.[73] This focus had a considerable amount to do with the fact that Rhode Island activists lacked a way of participating in issues of national importance. At the same time, ACT UP/RI's focus on privacy issues stemmed from the fact that Rhode Island activists possessed a less trusting relationship with state health officials than New York activists had experienced. As Michael K. Swirsky of ACT UP/New York's Testing and Disclosure Working Group noted, "In other states [besides New York], people don't see the health department as so benign. They see it much more as an enemy, and I think that's a reason why testing issues are much more a priority in certain areas of the country."[74]

Given its uneasy relationship with the Department of Health, then, ACT UP/RI devoted much of its activist energy to responding to state proposals for mandatory HIV testing and names reporting of people with HIV: in fact, one of ACT UP/RI's first actions—as well as its only action to involve civil disobedience—grew out of state Director of Health H. Denman Scott's active support for legislation allowing for certain forms of mandatory HIV testing.[75] ACT UP/RI also fought a continuous battle with the Rhode Island Department of Health over the availability of anonymous testing in the state, and in 1993, it organized around what were then already implemented state procedures requiring lab-based reporting to health officials of the names of people with low CD4+ counts.[76] Over time, ACT UP/RI settled into the role of a watchdog organization for the state: in addition to monitoring and demonstrating against the activities of the Department of Health, the group kept a close eye on the activities of private AIDS organizations such as Rhode Island Project/AIDS, the state's largest AIDS service organization.

ACT UP/RI's focus on these and other issues resulted in a number of important victories—victories that greatly improved the lives of people with HIV in the state. For instance, if ACT UP/RI had not campaigned vigilantly in favor of anonymous testing, the Rhode Island Department of Health would very likely have eliminated it altogether. At the same time, these victories, similar to the victories achieved by ACT UP/New York, were reformist in nature. State agencies and politicians altered their policies in response to ACT UP/RI, but these changes had little impact on the way in which either state government or even the Department of Health was run in general—nor were they intended to.

Moreover, focused as they were on local agencies and organizations, most of ACT UP/RI's activities had no impact whatsoever on people living outside of Rhode Island. Throughout its seven-year history, in fact, ACT UP/RI—as opposed to the larger New York chapter—was never really in a position to get at the "root" of problems related to AIDS, even if it had wanted to. AIDS is a problem of national (and international) proportions, and major interventions into the epidemic have had to be fought for at the national level. ACT UP/RI members did participate in a number of national ACT UP actions, and two of ACT UP/RI's founders (Stephen Gendin and James McGrath) divided their activist involvement between ACT UP/RI and ACT UP/New York. In addition, ACT UP/RI was an occasional participant in the ACT UP Network, a loose confederation of ACT UP chapters that would attempt to decide upon national strategy through the use of conference calls. Nonetheless, although much of ACT UP/New York's agenda was organized around large-scale problems such as the development of a cure or the federal AIDS definition, ACT UP/RI necessarily limited its focus to problems that were specific to Rhode Island.

TACTICS

Although almost everyone in ACT UP agreed on the goal of reform for most of its early history (if not as a general politics, then as a strategy appropriate to AIDS and ACT UP), the question of what tactics to pursue to achieve this goal was a much more controversial one—one which led to public fights and the exodus of certain groups from the organization. ACT UP is best known for the kinds of demonstrations I discussed earlier in this chapter—demonstrations that applied pressure to drug companies, bureaucrats, and politicians through street activism—all of which contribute to its militant reputation. As ACT UP members increasingly demonstrated both their knowledge about AIDS-related issues and their collective strength, however, opportunities for working on the inside—meeting with government officials, sitting on advisory boards at drug companies or in government agencies—became more frequent.[77] Accustomed to having and using access to powerful people and organizations as a way of getting what they wanted, white middle-class men in the organization proved especially willing to take advantage of such offers of a "place at the table."[78]

Soon, however, such an approach came under attack on two fronts. First, many activists argued that ACT UP's strength lay in its pushing from the "outside"—its street activism—or from meetings with officials that were backed up with actual or threatened demonstrations. Permanent positions on the "inside" actually managed to weaken ACT UP, they argued. Second, not only were white middle-class men more accustomed to using institutional access to achieve their goals, critics argued, they were also the only activists who were getting such access in the first place—in part because they were white men, and white men have more influence with people in power (most of whom are also white men themselves). And to the extent that many of the middle-class white men in ACT UP were more interested in and capable of advocating for the needs of people such as themselves, critics argued, the points of access they had cultivated were jeopardizing the ability of ACT UP members to advocate for the needs of other populations.[79]

This process was widely (and painfully) observed in ACT UP/ New York and has been discussed before. Nonetheless, the contribution I wish to make here in going over some of these debates again is to look at them as a central example of a division in approach within ACT UP that was grounded in the class style of different activists. Although commentators on these debates have generally argued that certain individuals were more inclined (or able) to work from the "inside" because they were white and male, I want to argue that this inclination also derived from the fact that such an approach was one with which middle-class men would have been more comfortable and familiar—in other words, that a particular class style was the overriding factor in these debates, rather than simply the mobilization of race and gender privilege (although, as we shall see, these played an unavoidable role as well). I also want to put an original spin on this discussion in two ways. First, other ways in which ACT UP's tactics were class driven will be discussed, including its heavy dependence on money and the limits that members put on the kinds of street activism that did occur. Second, by looking at a similar process that occurred in ACT UP/RI (although without the attendant debates), I hope to provide an analysis that has applications to other ACT UP chapters besides ACT UP/New York.

Inside and Out

Following an initial period in which street activism was the norm, both ACT UP/New York and ACT UP/RI experienced a similar shift in tactics: activist pressure in the form of demonstrations made opportunities to sit down with policymakers more available, and activists took eager advantage of them.[80] For many ACT UP/New York committees, such a shift meant that demonstrations would be increasingly combined with "inside" approaches whenever possible; peaceful negotiations and working on committees would be the preferred approach, and demonstrations would be resorted to when government and industry officials failed to see things in the same way as activists. In a 1992 pamphlet targeted at nonmembers, in fact, George Carter established such a combination approach—with the attendant assertion that activists were willing to negotiate and work with officials before resorting to demonstrations—as the official *modus operandi* of ACT UP. "This pamphlet" Carter explained:

> underscores the unseen side of ACT UP and highlights some of the subtler effects ACT UP has had. In addressing issues, an assessment is made of the problem and its impact. The problem is researched and studied—there is incredible expertise and experience in the ranks of ACT UP. Contact is made and, where possible, a resolution is achieved through talks. Frequently government, pharmaceutical or insurance companies maintain an air of arrogance or indifference. When all else fails, we take to the streets.[81]

Rank and file sentiment within ACT UP/New York supports Carter's assessment here. As Mark Golden discovered in 1992, a period of considerable infighting within ACT UP/New York over tactical issues, the vast majority of activists supported a combined "inside-outside" approach over the exclusive use of one or the other.[82]

For some committees, however, meeting with government and industry officials on the inside would almost entirely displace street activism as the preferred tactic for creating change. ACT UP/New York's Treatment and Data committee was one of the most prominent participants in ACT UP's overall movement away from street activism and toward working on the inside. Treatment and Data operated in a spotlight because the vast accumulated knowledge of drugs and drug trials that the members of T and D possessed provided the basis for many of ACT UP's demonstrations, as well as one of the reasons why government and industry officials proved increasingly willing to include activists in decision-making processes.[83] As T and D members began taking permanent positions on government committees, other activists criticized them for "selling out" or jeopardizing the work of the group as a whole. Eventually, any affiliation with an organization whose members might express reservations about the wisdom of taking permanent positions on the "inside" became too much for a number of prominent T and D members; in November 1991 these activists began leaving ACT UP to form what eventually became known as the Treatment Action Group (TAG). Although originally containing a street activist component, TAG eventually became a closed group of "experts," many of whom were paid. TAG's work relied almost exclusively on the extensive access to powerful government and industry officials they had cultivated, and its funding often came from pharmaceutical companies themselves.[84]

Similar to ACT UP/New York, ACT UP/RI experienced a shift away from street activism and toward meetings and negotiations—a shift that is symbolized by the group's movement from "art projects" to the Front Door Subcommittee, and from the Rocket to the Providence Center.[85] "Art projects" were acts of petty vandalism used to pressure (or even intimidate) public officials and to respond to public displays of homophobia: ACT UP/RI members used Christmas ornaments filled with paint to deface billboards trumpeting the campaigns of homophobic politicians or the products of antigay companies, replaced antigay or AIDS-phobic graffiti with more acceptable logos, and even spray painted slogans on the sidewalk outside of the home of Rhode Island Director of Health H. Denman Scott. Frequently adopted during the ACT UP/RI's early years, art projects (as well as other forms of street activism) were resorted to less often as government officials proved increasingly willing to meet with ACT UP members and as ACT UP/RI's membership made the gradual transition, in the words of Duncan A. Smith, away from a group with a "very 'street' sort of rough identity" to an organization with people "who are much more clued into the way bureaucracy works, and how you write a grant." Scott's replacement at the Rhode Island Department of Health, Barbara A. DeBuono, was fond of telling activists that she would be happy to meet with them any time if it would prevent a demonstration, and ACT UP members proved increasingly willing to take her and other state bureaucrats up on their offers.[86]

Eventually, the process of meeting with officials rather than demonstrating against them became so institutionalized that ACT UP/RI put together what became known as the Front Door Subcommittee. As its name suggests, the explicit purpose of the Front Door Subcommittee was to create change by approaching powerful individuals and organizations (politicians, health bureaucrats, the local AIDS service organization) by going through the front door—that is, through official channels. Activists made appointments, met with the appropriate people (often repeatedly), wrote polite and knowledgeable letters, and then, if all else failed (and people had the energy), organized a demonstration.

ACT UP/RI also experienced a change in membership makeup around 1990 that served to facilitate its movement from street activism to meetings with officials. "There are a lot more establishment-type people in ACT UP now than there were then," recalled Jesdale. "Then there were a lot more students, and lot more, sort of, people more on the fringe." Such a shift in membership, some activists felt, was itself enabled by a change in the location of the group's weekly meetings. In 1990, ACT UP/RI moved its meetings from the back room of the Rocket, a dance club, to the basement of the Providence Center, a social service agency, a change in venue that attracted certain kinds of people and discouraged others. "There's an ex-IDU [injection drug user] who's positive who just called me the other day," Jesdale noted, "and he said, 'You know, I went to two meetings at the Providence Center and I just couldn't go anymore.' He just didn't feel comfortable there at all."

To activists who joined ACT UP/RI after 1990, the push toward working from the "inside" was largely unnoticeable. But to those who had been with ACT UP/RI from the outset, the transformation in strategy could be astonishing. "I'm romantic for the days when we used to just sort of get together and do something," Jesdale indicated. The early ACT UP functioned on the notion that "you spray paint things on Denman Scott's sidewalk and call in a utility company to have his power shut off because you don't like him and you want him out of there," Jesdale explained. "You don't go about it by writing a letter to the governor or something—it didn't even occur to us to do stuff like that."

To a certain extent, working from the "inside" to achieve change was a tactic that made perfect sense in the context of an AIDS climate in which inside roles had opened up for people whose opinions had been previously excluded, and Rhode Island and New York activists of all stripes embraced this strategy to some extent or another. But although most ACT UP members saw the wisdom or logic of taking advantage of invitations to move to the bargaining table on occasion, the tendency of some ACT UP members and committees to do this to a point where other activists were actually outraged needs to be accounted for. Although ACT UP's move from the "outside" to the "inside" could be viewed as simply a strategic decision that could easily have gone the other way, I want to argue that this move was one that had been waiting to happen all along. Joining committees, dealing face-to-face with powerful officials, and taking a "place at the table," were moves that were entirely consistent with the class style that many of the men in both ACT UP/ New York and ACT UP/RI brought with them to those organizations. Such a tactical approach had proven impossible to adopt early in the history of ACT UP because bureaucrats and industry officials had simply been unwilling to negotiate with outsiders if they did not have to. Eventually, however, demonstrations and zaps forced these officials to open up dialogues with ACT UP, and male activists in particular—many of whom were highly accustomed to getting what they wanted by associating with powerful people—jumped at the long-awaited opportunity to move from the street to the conference room.

Not surprisingly, those committees that were predominantly composed of white middle-class men were the ones most likely to eschew street activism in favor of permanent positions on the inside. Treatment and Data in ACT UP/New York was one such committee. "The people who set the agenda for what strategies were going to be used in relation to treatments," Sarah Schulman (NYC) noted, "tended to be much more upper class, Ivy League educated, backgrounds in financial, investment." Although a number of committees focused on "treatment" issues in one form or another (ACT UP's various women's issues caucuses worked tirelessly on issues involving treatments for women), Treatment and Data was most noticeable in its move from the street to the conference table, in large part, I would argue, because working with people with power was a position that white middle-class men in particular were used to taking.

Certainly, Treatment and Data members were not allowed access to government officials just because they were white middle-class men; the impressive array of knowledge they possessed, combined with the activist movement they had behind them, undoubtedly played a much greater role in getting them access to government and industry players in the first place.[87] At the same time, these activists were more inclined to *accept* these inside positions—and to hold onto them even when they were not working—because as middle-class white men, they considered it more appropriate, more feasible, and ultimately more strategic (not to mention more familiar) to be working *with* those in positions of power rather than demonstrating against them. By contrast, possessing as they did an activist history in which they had always been on the "outside," many women in ACT UP remained skeptical about the advantages of working primarily from within.

Although T and D was perhaps the most prominent example of this shift from street activism to working from the inside, many of the ACT UP/New York members whom I spoke to in 1993 felt that the group as a whole had moved to a place similar to that which T and D occupied in 1991—replacing street activism with more accommodationist tactics. "I don't think there's even an understanding of using those two tactics together among a lot of people on the floor right now," ACT UP/New York member Trina Johnson told me. "I think a lot of people are just like, 'Let's write a letter, let's make a phone call,' and there's very few people who are remembering that you can use the meetings and the street together, a sort of one-two punch thing."

Of course, such an overall shift is not entirely surprising: although certain committees (such as T and D) were noticeable for the gender and class backgrounds of their members, ACT UP as a *whole* was always a majority white, middle-class, male organization. As such, although the class style of these men was most noticeable in committees such as T and D, it eventually came to dominate the entire organization. Activists themselves seemed vaguely aware of the class logic of this transformation. "I think ACT UP is a bunch of people who were nice boys and girls when they were growing up but don't really want to be too impolite," John Weir (NYC) explained, expressing frustration over ACT UP's tendency to opt for "diplomacy" over "abrupt agitation." Likewise, Johnson expressed concern over the energy and expectation many ACT UP members had invested in the 1992 presidential elections. "Sometimes I get a sense that people fall back," Johnson noted:

> that it's easy to go back to democratic [politics], or organizing around elections or candidates. . . . Working on the Bush/Clinton [election] last year was so acceptable to sort of white, middle-class, civic-minded gay people, and I think that has its place, but it's not what I want ACT UP to be focusing on now.[88]

ACT UP/RI's shift from street activism to working from the inside can be traced to a similar class logic, although local factors were important in this transformation as well. Whereas ACT UP/New York had certain committees that were made up predominantly of middle-class white men, ACT UP/RI was composed almost entirely of such men and had very few women and virtually no people of color for most of its history (ACT UP/RI's attempt to create a Women's Caucus in 1991 was short lived and highly controversial). If certain committees in ACT UP/New York were predisposed to move to negotiating from the inside, such a predisposition was evident in ACT UP/RI as a whole, especially after its membership shifted from mostly students to mostly professionals around 1990.

However, even though the class background of ACT UP/RI's membership is probably the most important reason why the group shifted its emphasis from street activism to negotiations, the political climate within which ACT UP/RI operated played an important role in this shift as well. ACT UP/RI members were even more likely than their counterparts in New York to feel that their group was perceived by outsiders as "radical," a perception that undoubtedly stemmed from the relatively conservative political climate of both the Rhode Island gay community and the state as a whole. This, in turn, tended to have a moderating effect on ACT UP/RI's activities—one that provided a considerable incentive for Rhode Island activists to replace street activism with negotiations once bureaucrats and politicians opened their doors to the group. "We let a lot of things go that perhaps we shouldn't let go," Alan Petrofsky (RI) explained. "But being in Rhode Island, things move a lot more slowly, and there's a lot less sympathy out there for some of the things that ACT UP stands for, and so we have to work within that system more." Moreover, as Genine Whitlock (RI) pointed out, in a "small state" such as Rhode Island, arrest and other forms of public protest were "less anonymous" than in a large city, discouraging extensive participation.[89] The class background of ACT UP/RI members was crucial to their decision to move to the conference table, then, but these local factors were also instrumental in pushing this process along.

Class privilege, of course, cannot be entirely separated from privileges stemming from race or gender. If the eagerness many men in ACT UP demonstrated upon being offered the opportunity to work from the inside can be traced to their class background, it is important to note that, at least in the minds of some activists, the fact that these men were also white and male played a considerable role in their receiving this opportunity in the first place. Even as male activists (largely from T and D) found themselves being offered permanent positions on advisory committees by government officials, women activists frequently found the same officials unwilling to listen to their concerns about the narrowness of the federal AIDS definition, the exclusion of women from government-sponsored trials, and other issues of particular importance to women. Whether actual or simply perceived, this discrepancy in treatment led to a series of heated debates within ACT UP/New York that threatened to tear the group apart.

As Cathy Cohen, among others, has noted, activists who were critical of the success that T and D members had in gaining access to government officials attributed much of this success to the fact that both the activists and the officials were white men.[90] Although male activists seemed to be having increasing success at influencing the opinions of government scientists and officials, women activists discovered that they were unable to get meetings with the same officials, or that when such meetings were granted, these officials proved unwilling to listen to them. During ACT UP's "Storm the NIH" demonstration in May of 1990, in fact, activists felt compelled to conduct a sit-in in the office of ACTG director Daniel Hoth in order to force him to meet with women in the group about women's issues, even though men in ACT UP had already been granted access to government scientists for some time.[91] When women in ACT UP did meet with government officials in July 1990, they were astonished to learn that these officials had an agreement with certain men in ACT UP that differences between ACT UP and themselves would be dealt with using polite negotiations, not demonstrations.[92] Besides contributing to a sense that women were being denied access to government officials simply because they were women, incidents such as these also led a number of ACT UP members to believe that T and D members were threatening the viability of ACT UP as a whole in their move to replace street activism with negotiations.

In some cases, these disagreements went public. Tensions erupted in the summer of 1990, for instance, over the decision by ACTG officials to provide activists, PWAs, and other "outsiders" with increased access to meetings and decision-making processes. For many activists, such increased access represented a significant development, given that the ACTG had the important responsibility of organizing AIDS drug trials for the federal government. In an article in *OutWeek* magazine, for instance, Mark Harrington expressed considerable enthusiasm over changes in the structure of the Ninth ACTG meeting in June 1990. That meeting, Harrington noted, represented "the first in which people with AIDS and activists were allowed to attend most sessions as official registrants," a shift in policy he attributed to ACT UP's massive "Storm the NIH" demonstration in May of that year.[93]

Other ACT UP members, however, expressed alarm at what they perceived to be certain activists' newfound insider status. Linda Meredith of ACT UP/DC, who also attended the Ninth ACTG meeting as an observer, wrote a response to Harrington's *OutWeek* article in which she expressed anger over what she viewed as the NIH's continued refusal to take seriously concerns related to women and HIV. Based on her observations at the meeting, Meredith maintained that "the answer for us, sisters, is still on the outside."[94] Tracy D. Morgan (NYC) expressed similar sentiments in a letter she also wrote in response to Harrington, chastising him for his enthusiasm over changes in ACTG procedures when so little had been proposed to address the NIH's inadequate research on women and AIDS. "Like it or not," Morgan informed Harrington, "you are quickly becoming a colleague of rational scientists in a position that many other activists do not occupy." Morgan then went on to accuse Harrington of having "sacrificed women" in order "to be accepted by this elite group."[95]

Not surprisingly, a number of prominent T and D members had a different interpretation of ACT UP's attempts to work with government scientists, and they refuted the wisdom of a political approach focused entirely on applying pressure from the outside. Writing in a 1991 opinion piece in the *Advocate*, for instance, T and D member Peter Staley questioned whether ACT UP had abandoned the "credo" of "by any means necessary" that he felt had proven successful in the group's early years. "If saving our lives . . . meant sitting down to a candlelight dinner with Tony Fauci . . . we'd do it," Staley explained. "If it meant kissing ass or kicking ass, we'd do it." Staley speculated, however, that the entrance into ACT UP of a number of individuals with "previous experience as social activists" had pushed the organization toward a new inflexible policy based more on idealism than pragmatism.[96]

Mark Harrington offered a similar criticism in an open letter written to ACT UP in March 1992. Harrington criticized what he termed "life-long 'movement activists'" who had begun objecting to inside roles for ACT UP members once rallies and demonstrations had finally forced government and industry officials to create such roles in the first place. Harrington pointed out the numerous successes ACT UP had experienced due to an " 'inside/outside' " strategy, and he argued that "these gains would have been impossible had we limited ourselves to the 'outside only' strategy favored by one faction within ACT UP."[97]

Not surprisingly, Harrington was especially critical of a small group of women activists who had proposed a "six-month moratorium on meetings with any government official about women's issues" early in 1991.[98] In making such a proposal, these women had come to the conclusion that women ACT UP members would never be given the kind of access to government scientists that the men in T and D possessed. As such, they argued, contact between ACT UP and government officials should be terminated (at least as concerned women's issues) so that these officials would not make the mistake of thinking that they were addressing all concerned parties in ACT UP by meeting with men from T and D.[99] B.C. Craig recalled the debate vividly. What certain activists were saying, Craig noted, was:

> "You don't care if women die; you only care if white gay men live, cause they're the only ones in trials, and the only ones being treated." . . . And the treatment activists said, "You think it's fine to go around acting like we're going to change the whole world when you have time to live for that, but I don't have time to live for that. Are you kidding? A six-month moratorium? I'll be dead before it's over: I'm dying, I need these drugs." . . . Each side was pointing their fingers at the other and saying, "You're killing me."

Debates such as these indicate the extent to which ACT UP's balancing act between street activism and inside access was closely intertwined with issues relating to the class, race, and gender identities of individual members. I have already outlined the extent to which these debates suggest the importance of a particular class style to ACT UP's adoption of a tactical strategy—a class style in which gaining access to powerful people was viewed as the optimal means of creating change. At the same time, the critiques of male activists which I have discussed here should remind us that the class style of male activists cannot be separated from their racial and gender identities. Presumably, the fact that many of the white men in ACT UP had had access to people in power before AIDS (especially when and if they chose to pass as straight) would have contributed to their overall commitment to the class style I have described—a commitment that would have been compromised (or at least put to the test) among women and people of color in ACT UP, despite their middle-class, professional backgrounds. In other words, white, middle-class gay men in ACT UP had a relationship to the dominant classes that was considerably less mediated than that of women and people of color in the group. Such a relationship came into play when certain activists were offered access to government officials and when these activists acted on the belief that taking advantage of these offers represented the optimal means of changing the government's response to AIDS.

ACT UP's gradual move over the years from street activism to working on the inside was not without its consequences. On the one hand, the access that both ACT UP/New York and ACT UP/RI were granted to health bureaucrats, politicians, and (in the case of ACT UP/New York) industry officials can be viewed as a positive development for the organization. ACT UP's move from the street to the conference table represented the materialization of one of the group's earliest demands—that people with AIDS and their advocates have as much of a say in AIDS policy as government scientists and industry officials. By moving to the "inside," ACT UP put itself in the position to contribute to the actual process of changing government and industry AIDS policy, rather than to simply make demands. Although demonstrations caused AIDS policymakers to realize that people were unhappy with their decisions in general, ACT UP's willingness to build on these demonstrations by meeting and working with officials was essential in getting these officials to adopt the specifics of ACT UP's proposals for change. As Garance Franke-Ruta noted in an interview conducted after ACT UP's "Storm the NIH" action, "The NIH action was more than just that one day down in Bethesda. The NIH action was months of work, and will continue to be months of work, because actions are used to open dialogue, and then we have to seize that dialogue."[100]

In many ways, however, ACT UP's move from the street to the conference table created more problems than it solved, as activists themselves were quick to note. B.C. Craig (NYC) summarized suc-cinctly what was perhaps the greatest concern among activists about working from the inside: "when they invite you in to sit down at the table," Craig noted, "they've neutralized you to some extent." Although Craig herself had no overall problem with ACT UP mem-bers meeting with government officials, she expressed concern over instances when such interactions became institutionalized, as when ACT UP members took permanent positions on government or industry advisory boards. "What happens," Craig explained:

> is once you get into that position, you're unwilling to give up that position, because that's the connection to your power. So, you speak out against something, but when it gets voted down, it's very difficult to walk out, because it means losing the power that you now believe that you have. And so we begin to focus on those positions as being our access points to power, instead of focusing on our street work as our access points to power.

Duncan A. Smith (RI) expressed a similar worry, noting that, after years of dealing with ACT UP, government agencies had devised a strategy of inviting activists in to negotiate as a means of neutralizing them:

> ACT UP is not, in my experience, equipped to do that. . . . we have no—other than going to the streets, or going to the media, which only works so much and no more—we don't have any leverage against that kind of thing. So they can make us a lot of promises and then just deliver nothing, and they know that.[101]

ACT UP members also worried that too much working from the inside could result in the loss of some of the advantages that went along with a broad-based, grassroots strategy. Activists pointed out, for instance, that working from the inside tended to limit the num-ber of people who could become actively involved in the organiza-tion. "People want to do something but they don't know how," Peter Hocking (RI) explained:

> and that's what I think ACT UP/RI and ACT UP nationally has been most successful at, is giving people some power, that

they've already had, but showing them how to use it. And when we get entrenched in the policy stuff, as important as it is, it's very difficult to keep those folks involved. Because they're not going to go to the meeting with [Providence mayor] Buddy Cianci, they're not going to go to a meeting with the governor's office staff people.

Smith expressed a similar concern, noting that ACT UP/RI's move toward institutionalization might have alienated members who were attracted to the group during its more direct action-oriented years.

Finally, ACT UP members expressed a concern that activism conducted behind closed doors could stifle the kinds of public protest that formed an important venue for the group's message. A demonstration "gets covered [by the press]," Bill Jesdale (RI) noted:

and it gets the conversation going, whereas going to the Health Department and talking with Mary Lou [DeCiantis][102] *again* doesn't raise any public discussion at all. It sort of keeps Mary Lou informed, it keeps us informed, but it doesn't generate any discussion of the issue in the public at large.[103]

Craig (NYC) expressed a similar concern about members taking permanent positions on the inside. "Often those meetings go with an articulated compromise: if we agree to this meeting, you won't have a protest. . . . And for a short period of time that's fine. . . . But when you go in and you sign on, you know, for some amount of time, that puts us all on hold."

As these comments—as well as the debates that I cited earlier in this section—indicate, activists in both ACT UP/RI and ACT UP/ New York experienced considerable unease over the consequences of the success both ACT UP chapters had in gaining access to policymakers. Even if such consequences could have been predicted, however, ACT UP's jump from the street to the conference table was a move that had been waiting to happen from the day that the group was founded. In the final analysis, ACT UP was comprised of professionals, not "radicals," and it is hardly surprising that as time went on "professional" conduct would gain ascendancy within the group. Many of the men in ACT UP did a very good job at posing as "militant," "radical" activists for as long as was necessary to secure a place at the conference table. Nonetheless, sitting at the table was the role that most of these men (and by extension ACT UP in general) were most comfortable with, adept at, and qualified to assume—a role that would not be abandoned (as we shall see) until internal divisions and the absence of a cure would push ACT UP in more radical directions later in its history.

Lawyers and Money

Although ACT UP/New York's willingness to work on the "inside" is probably the strongest evidence of the extent to which the class style of middle-class men came to dominate the group's tactics, other aspects of ACT UP/New York's operation point in a similar direction. ACT UP's heavy reliance on money is one such aspect. In a pattern that seems almost anomalous for a progressive, grassroots organization, ACT UP/New York proved almost entirely dependent for much of its history on large amounts of money to finance both major demonstrations and day-to-day operations—a dependence that turned into a crisis when money became scarce.

ACT UP/New York was famous for its fund-raising ability, earning amounts in a single night that could only be imagined by most grass-roots movements (ACT UP raised $300,000 from a celebrity art auction in 1989, $500,000 from another auction a year later, and tens of thousands from direct mail campaigns).[104] ACT UP/New York's ability to raise large amounts of cash to support its operations was tied to a number of factors, including the professional fund-raising experience that a number of members possessed and the connections that they had in business and art circles.[105] Most important, however, ACT UP had access to the incomes of its members and their friends, most of whom were financially secure gay men. "Now I'm in a lesbian organization, Lesbian Avengers," Sarah Schulman explained when I interviewed her in 1993, contrasting the financial situation of ACT UP and the Avengers:

> Our budget's about $15, because the fact of the matter is—and this was one of the things that was most impressive to me in many ways switching from the women's movement to the gay movement—men still earn twice as much as women in this country. And a gay men's movement is a movement of men's incomes. It has more discretionary income than any political movement I've ever seen in my life.

With money readily available, ACT UP/New York members became accustomed to a number of luxuries unavailable to other movements. In contrast to organizations that depended upon handmade signs, ACT UP owned a Xerox machine that took up an entire room, that could mass produce professional-looking graphics and posters, and that cost $10,000 a month to lease. Unlike movements that were accustomed to herding their members into buses and caravans, ACT UP was frequently able to fly its members to conferences and demonstrations and put them up in hotels once they arrived.[106] ACT UP/New York rented a "work space" on West 29th street for $2,000 a month, and its budget for demonstrations was immense—$83,000 alone for the International Conference on AIDS in San Francisco in 1990, money that went to setting up an elaborate communications center with fax machines and computers.[107] Unable to buy themselves a cure for AIDS, ACT UP members proved quite capable of buying themselves anything else they felt was necessary for the fight that could eventually bring that cure about.

Because of ACT UP/New York's dependence on large amounts of money, however, the group found its ability to function—as well as its identity as an organization—severely threatened when funds became dangerously low in 1993.[108] ACT UP/New York's expenses exceeded its income by almost $54,000 in the first quarter of 1993, and even with increased income in the second quarter of that year, the deficit for 1993 remained at approximately $25,000. ACT UP had been able to draw from its reserve in order to save itself from bankruptcy, but by the summer of 1993, the reserve had dipped to the dangerously low level of $13,000.[109]

Nonetheless, even in the face of these dire conditions, ACT UP continued to approve spending requests at the levels it had done during the boom years when massive art auctions had filled its coffers:[110] not only were members unwilling to adopt levels of spending commensurate with the amount of money that was on hand, they seemed unable even to imagine how ACT UP could function without large amounts of money.[111] Having just managed to get back on its feet after the departure of a number of prominent activists to form TAG, T and D members in particular bristled at the idea that their day-to-day operating expenses would have to be approved by the entire floor under a proposed emergency plan. "It is very important for Treatment and

Data to have security in terms of funds," T and D member Carlos Maldonado (NYC) told me:

> because there are a lot of conferences, and like I said, the activism now has changed more into, you have to go to these places, you have to talk to these researchers, you have to influence the protocols, you have to really get all these tools to deal with these people. And in order to do that, you have to spend money.

As Maldonado's comment here indicates, in the minds of many activists, access to those individuals in the position to make important AIDS-related decisions was closely tied to ACT UP's ability to spend money. Although ACT UP was not in the position to buy influence, it viewed its ability to function at the same level as those in government and industry (flying to conferences, producing professional-looking documents, etc.) as essential to its ability to influence these sectors.

ACT UP's perceived need to be able to operate at the level of government and industry officials cannot entirely explain its dependence on money—and its terror at not having it anymore—for ACT UP believed it essential to bankroll its street activism as much as its negotiations. Certainly, the level of denial that ACT UP members demonstrated concerning spending can be attributed, in part, to the fact that members had become accustomed to ACT UP's functioning in a certain way over a several-year period. At the same time, this unwillingness to curtail spending (or even to imagine curtailing spending) on the part of many members might also be attributed to the fact that most of these activists did not have to operate under similar austerity measures in either their workplace environments or their personal lives. Business people would have to take the bottom line into account when making managerial decisions, of course, but the idea that photocopying, making long-distance phone calls, or flying to meetings might have to be reduced or eliminated was an unimaginable concept to male activists in particular, many of whom had extensive experience with the realities of the business world but little previous background in grassroots organizing. Just as the access that individual ACT UP members had to money in their personal and business lives had caused ACT UP to adopt an operating style that relied on a steady flow of cash, the class backgrounds of members created a situation in which functioning as an activist movement without large amounts of money—a situation that most progressive movements in this country have taken for granted—became simply unimaginable later on.[112]

The limits that ACT UP put on its street activism provides another example of the extent to which ACT UP's middle-class orientation influenced its tactics. Although many activists perceived ACT UP's demonstrations as a "radical" alternative to the negotiations and committee assignments that were increasingly consuming the group's energies, ACT UP's street activism can best be understood as what I would call "bourgeois militancy." On the one hand, the financial resources that both individual activists and the group as a whole possessed allowed ACT UP to engage regularly in the kinds of militant protests that poor people are able to resort to in only the most exceptional of circumstances.[113] On the other hand, in contrast to the activist movements that *have* occurred among poor people in this country (the Civil Rights movement of the 1950s and 1960s being one prominent example), ACT UP took its street activism only so far as was comfortable for a group of middle-class activists with professional jobs. Demonstrations were planned that would attract significant media attention, but ACT UP/New York members—along with their Rhode Island counterparts—tended to avoid activities that could result in serious or long-term punishment or jeopardize people's careers. As Stephen Gendin (NYC/RI) noted, for instance, many ACT UP/New York members exhibited considerable discomfort when Larry Kramer began advocating the use of violence. "These are all people who have jobs and things like that," Gendin explained, "and they don't want to get arrested for blowing up a building." At the same time, Gendin suggested, the class position of these activists created a situation in which individuals were able to get arrested in the first place: "they'd be perfectly happy to get arrested for a CD [civil disobedience] especially when they know from their hot-shot lawyers . . . that what they're going to do is pay a $50 fine or a $100 fine, and they're making $50,000."

B.C. Craig (NYC) echoed Gendin's sentiment, viewing ACT UP as representing a significant departure from the kinds of grassroots organizations with which she had worked previously—groups in which getting arrested generally meant that "you stay in jail until they throw you out." Although most of the members of these organizations "did work that they considered to be less important than the activist work they did, so they were constantly taking off time and being away for stretches of time, and losing jobs and taking new jobs," ACT UP members (especially later in the group's history) had a very different relationship to their activism. "People have real jobs where they make real money, and they don't take off a lot of time. . . ," Craig noted. "And people expect in ACT UP to be out of jail that day so that they can sort of resume their life the next day." As these comments indicate, even when certain activists advocated having ACT UP eschew the kinds of access that it had managed to cultivate and return to the street activism for which it was best known, the street activism that these ACT UP members promoted was also a distinctly middle-class form of protest. In other words, whatever tactics it adopted in a particular situation, ACT UP was never able to stray very far from its class origins.

EPILOGUE

The years 1991 through 1993 witnessed two important developments for ACT UP: a nationwide perception that the group was on the decline and ACT UP's work around universal health care and the Barbara McClintock Project to Cure AIDS. As a wrap-up to my study of ACT UP, I want to consider the ways in which these two developments symbolized ACT UP's eventual coming to terms with the limits of a reform approach.

ACT UP/New York's troubles during this period were widely rehearsed in both gay and mainstream media sources, and they weighed heavily on the minds of most long-term members when I conducted my fieldwork in the summer of 1993.[114] The departure of key Treatment and Data Committee members to form the Treatment Action Group beginning in 1991, a precipitous decline in membership and in the level of activity among those who did stay involved, the deaths of a number of prominent activists, a decrease in high-visibility initiatives, a sense of dislocation with the election of a seemingly sympathetic Democratic president, and the budget crisis of 1993 all contributed to a growing perception that ACT UP/ New York was facing serious problems.[115]

ACT UP/RI had its share of problems during this period as well. Rhode Island activists—especially those who had been around since the early days of the organization—experienced the downside to ACT UP/RI's increased professionalization—the loss of the ability to mobilize quickly and effectively that had been the hallmark of the group's younger self. Although numbers in ACT UP/RI had remained stable and finances were actually up, the energy and spontaneity that had previously infused the group seemed lost, according to members.

Undoubtedly, the infighting and personal attacks endemic to leaderless movements had something to do with the exodus from ACT UP chapters nationwide. As Craig (NYC) noted, "We're all humans, and so there's an enormous amount of backbiting, and jealousy, and personal attacks that makes you feel like, 'Why am I wasting my time? I would be better off being a buddy or doing service work.'" But even more centrally, the loss of membership and energy within ACT UP— and ACT UP/New York in specific—might be understood in terms of both the successes and failures of a reform approach.[116]

On one level, members suggested, a decrease in the number of people willing to devote time to ACT UP/New York stemmed from the palpable successes that AIDS activists had experienced over the previous few years. "The most optimistic thing you could say," Michael Swirsky remarked in relation to ACT UP's decline, "is maybe it's a victim of its own success. . . . Perhaps people feel it has achieved its purpose." Stephen Gendin, a once extremely active member who had left ACT UP by the time I interviewed him, sounded a similar note. "Anger and things like that come in waves," Gendin explained:

. . . . I think when people thought that ACT UP did some initial good, the anger sort of dispersed, HIV became a much more acceptable thing to talk about, and people felt less isolated. . . . [P]eople started feeling like they could become social again, and that dissipates the energy of feeling like you have to spend every minute of your life doing ACT UP stuff, which is sort of how I felt for a couple of years, and how most of the people I was associating with felt.

As these remarks suggest, ACT UP's tendency to concentrate on limited reforms might have eventually contributed to its own decline. By conceptualizing its activist mission as a series of short-term, winnable battles, ACT UP unwittingly created a situation in which a number of activists believed that, once those battles had been successfully won, a cure was around the corner and their work was done.

Ironically, however, the *limits* of such a reform approach—that it did not and perhaps could not produce a cure—drove other members away as well. Many activists who had originally joined ACT UP/ New York in the belief that it would be the best way to save their own lives or the lives of friends became discouraged with the realization that piecemeal reforms would not be enough, that the level of commitment needed to produce a cure would be considerably greater than they had originally anticipated. "I think that in 1987," Swirsky explained:

> people might have been a little more naive. I think there were people who really thought that a cure could be had by screaming and yelling. And ACT UP certainly revealed, and helped to correct, a lot of deficiencies in the way that drugs are produced and tested, of course. . . . I think though . . . that people realize a cure is not going to come around the corner. . . . And I think that reality has hit people very hard, or has hit people hard gradually over the course of the past several years. And I think people have been turning away from ACT UP because of the length of the fight and because of the difficulty.

Jon Winkleman provided a similar explanation of why he had decided to take a leave from ACT UP/New York at the time I spoke to him. "Emotionally, I just need a break," Winkleman said:

> One of the reasons I became involved is because some people I know are very ill, and I initially thought that, if I get involved, we can save their lives. And I think I'm coming to the conclusion that those aren't the lives that I'm going to save, that my friends who matter the most to me are going to die, and it's not within my power to change that. I think that's one of the heavy things weighing on all of ACT UP right now.

"People need time to emotionally regroup," Winkleman indicated, a process that involved members trying to create a space for the grief that accompanied the anger they usually showed.[117]

Nonetheless, in response to the realization that incremental reforms would be inadequate to the task of rapidly producing a cure, ACT UP mobilized around a more radical solution—the Barbara McClintock Project to Cure AIDS. Named after the Nobel Prize–winning scientist who adopted unconventional research methods for her work on DNA, the McClintock Project constituted ACT UP's blueprint for the kind of AIDS "Manhattan Project" promised by Bill Clinton during his presidential campaign.[118] In short, the McClintock Project was geared toward a fundamental restructuring of the way basic AIDS research (or any medical research) is performed in this country. It aimed at eliminating the extensive conflicts of interest endemic to medical research conducted within a market economy, as well as at nurturing AIDS-related theories excluded by dominant research paradigms. By organizing basic AIDS research into a centralized, federally funded program, the McClintock Project, according to its creators, was intended to eliminate a number of problems hampering such work: the "corporate domination of research agenda" (e.g., drug company influence over research priorities); the monolithic focus on theories of viral (or single viral) origins for AIDS (a focus driven in part by the reality that viral science is currently highly prestigious—and consequently brings in the most grants); and uncoordinated and competitive research, which leads to extremely limited communication between different kinds of scientists.

The McClintock Project was designed to address these problems by providing a central location for most federally funded AIDS research and by prohibiting conflicts of interests among researchers stemming from affiliations with "universities, pharmaceutical companies, private research organizations, etc." All results from the Project would be made readily available to other researchers and members of the general public, and companies and individuals alike would be prohibited from experiencing "financial gain" from "curatives" developed by the Project. Finally, the Project would be granted eminent domain over drugs and other research results produced by non-McClintock institutions.

In a number of ways, the McClintock project represented a truly radical—or "root"—solution to the problems blocking the development of a cure for AIDS. In the first place, it constituted a fundamental reconceptualization of the way in which medical research is conducted in the United States, in that it divorced AIDS research from financial gain for drug companies and professional advancement for scientists. By scrapping the NIH practice of giving drugs discovered through government-funded research to private companies for production and marketing, and by allowing control of a drug to be taken away from a company if it delayed production for financial reasons for an excessive amount of time, the McClintock Project represented a fundamental challenge to market paradigms for scientific research. Second, the Project allowed for more inquiry into the root causes of AIDS by opening up pathogenesis research to a variety of theories currently ignored. Finally, and most important, although most medical research in this country was and is focused on developing alleviatives for symptoms, the McClintock Project was intended to produce a cure.

The McClintock Project was in fact so sweeping—and so fundamentally different from the way science is conducted—that it proved controversial across the board. The Project received a lukewarm response from White House AIDS Coordinator Kristine Gebbie, and even activists themselves disagreed about its merits. "The idea of a Manhattan Project for what's been lumped as basic research is criticized—even by AIDS activists I know, or people who have been in ACT UP—as ridiculous, because basic research 'just ain't done that way,'" Swirsky remarked. Doubts were even expressed within the ranks of ACT UP's recently revitalized Treatment and Data Committee over certain provisions of the McClintock Project. "Some people in T and D felt it was ridiculous," Kevin Robert Frost (NYC) explained:

> to expect that a capitalist government was suddenly going to take away patents from companies, or even to suspect that this government for the first time would even have people's interests at heart rather than business' interests at heart. Never has been that way, I think it's not ever going to be that way in a capitalist society, and so there were those that felt it wasn't worth investing the effort into that, and those that felt it was.

In many ways, the McClintock Project represented a move in a new direction for ACT UP. Sweeping proposals for structural change were relatively unusual for ACT UP—a group that members indicated had historically been more comfortable with counteracting government and industry mistakes rather than with producing solutions of its own, and that tackled epidemiological problems more through "minutia" than through the development of broad-based proposals.[119] As such, the McClintock Project constituted one of ACT UP's first real attempts to develop a radical solution for ending AIDS, rather than merely arguing that radical changes (end racism, end poverty) might be needed but focusing on more winnable battles instead.

The McClintock project was not the only radical approach to ending AIDS that ACT UP endorsed in the early 1990s. ACT UP's work around universal health care represented the flip side of its development of the McClintock Project: if the McClintock Project represented a radical program for developing a cure for AIDS, universal health care constituted a radical approach to the delivery of this cure to those who needed it. For ACT UP, universal health care went to the root of the problems surrounding health care delivery in the United States—millions of Americans lacked access to quality health care because they had no health insurance. Although ACT UP had previously concentrated on trying to reform the practices of individual insurance companies that were discriminating against PWAs, beginning in 1991, it expanded its approach to the problem of health care delivery by joining a coalition of progressive organizations pushing for the establishment of universal health care in the United States.[120]

ACT UP's involvement in the issue of universal health care crystallized in October 1991, with a demonstration in Washington, DC, organized by the ACT UP Network.[121] Writing in a handbook put together to accompany the event, demonstration organizers came to the conclusion that, in its attempts to address the day-by-day emergencies that AIDS produces, ACT UP had failed to consider more radical responses to the epidemic. "We have had to fight battle after battle for immediate, stopgap measures just to keep people *alive*. Our targets sometimes seemed scattered. . . . We have not taken the time nor devoted the energy to long-term goals or broad-based solutions," one article in the handbook argued.[122] Drawing on the energy from the demonstration, ACT UP helped to put the spotlight on national health care during the 1992 presidential campaign, and when the Clinton administration began devising a plan to present to Congress for a national health care program, ACT UP joined other coalition members in demanding a single-payer plan modeled after the Canadian system.[123]

In endorsing a single-payer plan, ACT UP contributed to a fundamental critique of the capitalist nature of the health care system in the United States, in which health care delivery is understood as a for-profit venture. Moreover, in insisting that a cure should be available to anyone who needed it, regardless of ability to pay, ACT UP put a radical spin on the crisis of consumption that had motivated many men to join the group in the first place. Although the inability of middle-class gay men with plenty of disposable income to purchase a drug that could save their lives was still viewed a crisis in itself, the fact that most PWAs could not afford a cure even if it existed was increasingly viewed as a crisis as well.

ACT UP's critique of capitalism would be repeated in its development of the McClintock Project, and it served to distance ACT UP considerably from its previous reformist approach. After a number of years in which the backgrounds of members led them to believe that minor reforms in government and industry would be enough to address the needs of PWAs, the limits of such a position became painfully evident in the early 1990s. In contrast to an approach in which drug companies, insurance companies, and individual government agencies were envisioned as permanent entities that would have to be worked with (or at least tolerated), ACT UP's endorsement of both universal health care and the McClintock Project constituted fundamental assaults on as deeply entrenched an institution as American capitalism. Late in its existence, ACT UP devised a radical agenda for a crisis that was clearly not to be ended by reform, and common perceptions of ACT UP as a radical organization began to prove true at last.

Chapter 2

Consumption and Cure: Paul Monette, Larry Kramer, Sarah Schulman

"ALL THEY NEEDED": PAUL MONETTE'S AFTERLIFE

Money can't buy you love. It also can't buy you a cure for AIDS. In Paul Monette's 1990 novel *Afterlife,* protagonists Mark Inman and Steven Shaw are in desperate need of both: the love relationship that could save their emotional lives and the cure that could rescue them from death. But as with many of the gay men I have just discussed who were driven into activism for the first time, Mark and Steven live in a world in which not everything that is needed can simply be bought.[1]

Although Mark and Steven are not activists, *Afterlife* represents a useful text with which to follow my analysis of ACT UP because the issues of class and consumption that shaped that organization are structuring influences in the novel as well. As I have already discussed, affluent gay men discovered in AIDS a problem whose solution was not for sale, and in many cities, this crisis of consumption drove hundreds of them into grassroots activism. Paul Monette was among these men. As he describes in his 1988 memoir *Borrowed Time,* the 1985 AIDS diagnosis of his lover Roger completely shattered the privileged life the couple had built for themselves in Los Angeles.[2] Monette became involved with ACT UP, serving as a press liaison (along with film historian Vito Russo) at its "Seize the FDA" demonstration in 1988. He wrote a fund-raising letter for the local chapter of ACT UP in Los Angeles, and he included an ACT UP demonstration in the "AIDS" episode of *Thirtysomething* he was commissioned to write (the scene was later excised).[3]

By employing the medium of fiction, however, Monette was able to "resolve" this crisis of consumption along very different lines. Mark and Steven, similar to their real-life counterparts, come to realize the limits of consumption. But although such a realization drove many gay men into activism, Mark and Steven's realization drives them away from commodities and into each other's arms.

Afterlife tells the story of three Los Angeles AIDS "widowers" who had met each other in a hospital while their respective lovers were dying and have formed an informal support group since: Steven Shaw, the owner of a travel agency he has not entered since the death of his partner; Dell Espinoza, a Mexican immigrant who owns a landscaping company; and Sonny Cevathas, a New Age enthusiast. Although *Afterlife* purports to give equal attention to the stories of these three men, Steven Shaw is really the main protagonist of the novel, and as with many literary protagonists, his central task is to overcome the forces that have kept him from falling in love again. Steven eventually meets Mark Inman, a television executive who has recently discovered that he himself is HIV positive. The lovers-to-be face some of the usual stumbling blocks—undelivered phone messages, misunderstood signals, and most important, Steven's grief at the loss of his previous partner—as well as some unusual situations, including Steven's discovery of Mark having sex with Sonny. Nonetheless, with everyone around them giving the embryonic relationship their emphatic blessing (and often at the most unlikely of moments), Steven's and Mark's ability to resist falling in love ultimately crumbles. Steven's co-worker Margaret predicts as early as the Thanksgiving dinner at which Mark and Steven admit their love for each other that everything will turn out "happily ever after,"[4] and by the end of the novel, she has been proven correct.

As much as it is a novel about love, however, *Afterlife* is a novel structured by anxieties about consumption. Highly affluent themselves, Mark and Steven live in a world in which material objects exist in excess and everyone can seemingly afford whatever they want. Characters in *Afterlife* are surrounded by commodities, and they evaluate one another based on ownership and consumption. Monette drops expensive product names throughout his novel—Armani and Polo; Bentley, Porsche, Ferrari, and Volvo; Wedgwood teacups; and Porthault sheets. Arriving at Mark's house for the first time, an embarrassed Steven averts his eyes from Mark, concentrating on the expensive interior of the house instead: "terra-cotta floor scattered with Indian rugs" (pp. 79-80), a sofa that Steven guesses to be "Finnish, about four grand" (p. 80). Sonny, another AIDS widower, takes this process of evaluation one step further, searching for the lover who is wealthy enough to return him to the splendors of an imagined past life among the Pharaohs. Sonny may not understand his new lover Sean Pfieffer's business dealings, we learn, but "the money he understood . . . and the post-mod house at the top of Trousdale, commanding a two-seventy view of the glittering prizes" (p. 185).

The pinnacles of consumption in *Afterlife,* however, are Lou Ciotta and his wife Angela. Lou is a multimillionaire sitcom star whose salability (contracts, product endorsements) constitutes Mark's full-time job. Lou and Angela are new to money, and they consume with a passion as a result. Early in the novel, Lou calls Mark wanting to buy a horse for "a million two" (p. 37), refusing to listen to his lawyer's plea that the Ciotta household "can't afford it." "I don't want to hear that shit," Lou bellows. "It's all I ever heard growin' up" (p. 42). Angela, a former Miss Arizona, is just the same, "shop[ping] with a murderous vengeance day after day" (p. 38) (as with the noblewomen at the Court of Versailles, Angela is forbidden from wearing the same dress twice). Angela and Lou live in a "Norman Chateau" that formerly belonged to Gary Cooper, and Angela has so many clothes in her room-sized closet that she has nothing to do but "give it away like crazy. My sisters, my old girlfriends—they leave here with both arms full. I'm like Santa Claus" (p. 116). The Ciotta's consumption frenzy invades Mark's house as well. When Mark quits working for Lou suddenly, Lou attempts to woo him back using the language most familiar to the two men—commodities:

> "Look at all the shit he sends me," Mark declared with contempt. "I feel like a fuckin' game show."
> He waved across the room toward an improbable clutter of toys: a stationary bicycle, a VCR, a stork-like Italian desk lamp, a video camera, a telescope, all heaped by the window as if waiting for a Christmas tree. This was the booty with which Lou Ciotta was trying to woo Mark Inman back to work. A new gift arrived every third day. (p. 80)

Consumption appears in *Afterlife* in another form as well—conspicuous and recurrent eating. Dates take place at restaurants, and Steven has taken up food as a hobby, gaining twenty-five pounds since his partner Victor died. Steven gobbles up Chips Ahoy cookies and a Mud Pie before even two paragraphs of the novel have transpired, and paragraph two of *Afterlife* describes all of his needs in terms of the food he does not have on hand: "Steven had no beer; he had no salad; no milk for the coffee; no peanuts; no bread. And seven people were coming in half an hour" (p. 2). Eating as a form of consumption functions on a metaphoric level as well: when Mark shows up at Steven's door, an uninvited guest for the widower's dinner, Steven recalls him as someone who "eats gorgeous men for breakfast" (p. 10).

But if conspicuous consumption is a way of life in the world that Steven and Mark live in, both men (and even Angela Ciotta) learn the lesson that AIDS has taught to affluent gay men—that money cannot always buy everything one needs. Facing a problem that cannot be resolved with a purchase, Mark and Steven's faith in the power of consumption reaches a point of crisis—a moment in which the promise of the commodity to satisfy all needs is shown to be a lie and the limits of the marketplace are made painfully clear.[5] As such, both men find themselves repelled by the commodities they valued so strongly while healthy. Steven's ownership of a travel agency—and his unlimited access to all the corners of the world—means nothing to him now that Victor is dead. "Shaw Travel mocked him now with all its promise of freedom," he realizes, "the paradise beaches and Gold Card souvenirs. For Steven travel was over" (p. 9). Mark is described in similar terms, disenchanted with the material rewards of working for Lou. "Though he had enough perks to choke a horse—car phone, half-acre granite desk, personal trainer—he'd just had a whole day of being abandoned and unloved" (p. 12), and Mark expresses "contempt" for the "shit" that Lou sends to woo him back (p. 80). Mark, in fact, quits his job while talking on the phone with Lou, pushed over the edge by Lou's incessant babble about the money he is making and what he wants to buy—things that mean little to Mark anymore. Consumption is for the healthy, not the dying. Mark and Steven realize this while watching Christmas shoppers on the news, a lesson that is also made clear when the two men pile their friend Ray Lee's now useless possessions out on the curb after Ray has died from AIDS. Even Angela Ciotta demonstrates a final frustration with consumption, leaving Lou and his million-dollar act to start a new life.[6]

Early in *Afterlife,* after his dinner guests have left, an exasperated Steven talks aloud to his deceased partner Victor in an attempt to determine what he "needs" in life, and Steven's elliptical inquiry serves as the underlying question for the entire novel:

> "I can't take care of them anymore," he said, meaning Dell and Sonny. There was no sign of protest. "I need . . ." he continued tentatively. "I need to . . ." But he quickly fizzled out, stumped for a verb, as if he couldn't translate fast enough from another tongue. He stared into the living room, where the gas fire still rippled in the fireplace. His party had vanished like a parlor trick. There was no more mud in the freezer. He couldn't even imagine what he needed. (p. 20; ellipses in original)

Steven's inquiry as to what he "needs" is echoed later in the novel as well. As Steven leaves Mark's house after his initial visit, Mark offers him a present from the booty pile that Lou has sent over. "Here, take something," Mark tells Steven. "Mark walked over to the corner full of treasure, hugging himself excitedly. 'You need a camera? You want this lamp?'" (p. 88). And when Steven's co-worker Margaret intrudes upon Mark and Steven kissing as she searches for an item for their Thanksgiving dinner, Steven responds to the invasion by rephrasing the question he posed early in the novel. "What do we need?" (p. 217) he asks his startled guest, the "we" referring literally to Margaret, but metaphorically to the two men.

What Mark and Steven need (and cannot buy), of course, is a magic bullet cure for AIDS, something that Mark learns during his business trip to Europe is not waiting in the wings in 1987, the year that *Afterlife* takes place. Committed to writing a novel faithful to the experiences of HIV-positive men, but simultaneously committed to his "happily ever after" ending, Monette, like Steven, cannot articulate what HIV-positive men really need—a cure—for there are no happy endings to be had in 1987 as far as a cure for AIDS is concerned. Instead, I would argue, Monette relegates this *unresolvable* crisis of consumption to the margins of his novel, focusing on a *resolvable* crisis of consumption in its place: Mark and Steven's frustrations with consumption are still shown to stem from a realization that what they need cannot be bought, but it is love, rather than a cure, that is missing from their lives. In contrast to the unavailability of a cure, however, this particular crisis of consumption is easily resolved through the union of the two men. Both men learn to value love over things, for although Mark and (to a lesser extent) Steven have everything money can buy, "everything," they come to learn, does not include love.

As I suggested earlier, both men have considerable trouble with the courtship process, as they are used to fulfilling their needs with the simple flash of a credit card, and their difficulties provide the plot twists that give *Afterlife* much of its shape. Minor characters in the novel show Mark and Steven the way, however: although no one in *Afterlife* suggests that fighting for a cure might help Mark and Steven get what they need, everyone points to the importance of finding a partner. Reminded by such people as Mark's father that "everything else [besides love] is shit" (p. 178), Mark and Steven succeed in their quest, bonded by the end of the novel. In effect, then, what Mark and Steven do is to "defetishize" the commodity, evacuating its false promise and reinvesting this promise in romantic love. With nothing available for purchase that could save their lives, love, rather than the commodity, becomes that which is "transcendent."[7]

One reason why a love plot is so central to *Afterlife*, then, is because it allows Monette to acknowledge the inability of the commodity to meet the AIDS-related needs of affluent gay men while simultaneously offering a "resolution" for the crisis of consumption that has occurred as a result. Love in *Afterlife* acts as a stand-in for a cure—in more ways than one. First, in having Mark and Steven find love—in resolving one kind of crisis stemming from the limits of what money can buy—Monette can provide a metaphoric resolution for the fact that an AIDS cure would elude a generation of gay men. Second, by framing Mark and Steven's union as a utopian fantasy, one which promises to shut out disease and death, Monette is able to salvage the utopian promise that is normally invested in the commodity, but whose illusory nature was evidenced for gay men with the arrival of AIDS. *Afterlife* is still able to come to a utopian ending, but it is love rather than commodities that brings this about.

By working through a love story, moreover, Monette is able to resolve this crisis of consumption while maintaining the plausibility of the story he tells, thereby remaining at least somewhat faithful to the historical situation of gay men. Monette could have introduced a cure into his book, but such a "solution" to Mark and Steven's problems would have rung extremely false in a novel set in 1987. "The sleepers had all they needed" (p. 278), Monette writes in the paragraph that ends the novel, so that love becomes the answer to Steven's elliptical inquiry at the beginning of the novel as to what he "needs." A cure for their infection may never be found, but the lovers have "all they needed" nonetheless.

A second and related reason why Monette affords the love plot in *Afterlife* so much weight stems from the relationship that "happily ever after" love stories have to all that gay men have lost to AIDS—including, as I argued earlier, the tentative positioning that many gay men had within the dominant classes. Since one thing that AIDS has taken away from many gay men is, in fact, their lovers, a love story provides a useful way to suggest the return to gay men of their former lives. Mark and Steven's union functions as a reminder of a time before AIDS, when love between men could lead to "happily ever after" instead of death and loss. By giving Steven a new partner, Monette returns to Steven his life situation before his partner Victor got sick—in other words, before the epidemic. Mark's health status (HIV-positive, but no signs of sickness) is extremely important in this regard, for although Steven and Victor had continued their travels around the world as long as Victor's lesions were hidden by his clothes, the two men "never went any-where again" after Victor discovers a lesion below his ear (p. 23). By concluding his novel before either Mark or Steven get sick themselves, then, Monette is able to evoke the circumstances of a pre-AIDS gay relationship, one unaffected by death and disease. In fact, in one important respect (the *most* important respect), life is even better for Mark than it was before AIDS, since meeting Steven has caused him to realize the importance of falling in love.

Questions of plausibility are crucial here as well, for the happily resolved love story allows Monette to suggest the return to gay men of their lives before AIDS without undermining the realistic nature of his novel. Monette would have been hard pressed to depict two

HIV-positive men recovering all aspects of their pre-AIDS lives in a novel set in 1987, and in fact, both men's lives take major turns for the worse because of the epidemic (while Steven loses his partner to AIDS, Mark quits his job upon learning he is sick and is denied disability payments). By contrast, Mark and Steven's union is perceived as a plausible (and even predictable) ending to the novel, allowing it to act as a metaphor for a more general recovery of all that gay men have lost to AIDS.[8]

Unlike Mark and Steven, Dell, another of the AIDS widowers, never finds another partner, but his fate in the novel is also intertwined with the crisis of consumption I have just described. While Mark and Steven spend their time falling in love, Dell channels his anger into political struggle. Dell becomes a one-man activist/terrorist hit squad as the novel progresses: he falsely informs the local water department that he has contaminated a reservoir with HIV-infected blood, setting off the predicted panic; he pours turkey blood throughout the office of Mother Evangeline, a right-wing preacher who sees AIDS as God's retribution against homosexuals; and in the final scenes of the novel, he blows Mother Evangeline's head off live on cable television and then kills himself.

Dell's violent ending—as well as his activist role—stems from his own relation to issues of class and consumption: because Dell is Chicano and a manual worker, he is unable to participate in the recuperative ending that Monette envisions for men such as Mark and Steven. Affluent gay men experienced AIDS as a crisis of consumption because it gave the lie to their previous ability to purchase whatever they needed or wanted; Dell, by contrast, is a Mexican immigrant, a man for whom such powers of consumption have always been a distant dream. Likewise, by marking them as gay and stealing their health, AIDS undermined the ability of gay white men to pass as straight, thereby dislodging their already tentative hold within the dominant classes; an immigrant, a Chicano, and a man who speaks with an accent, Dell, by contrast, has been marked as "other" since long before the epidemic began. Removed from the classes of gay men for whom AIDS represented a form of class dislocation, and for whom "happily ever after" would be a genuine possibility were the epidemic to end, Dell's problems cannot be resolved by the conclusion of the novel. Fittingly, then, Dell refuses to look for another lover after the death of his partner Marcus, disqualifying himself from the metaphoric resolutions that romantic love offers to men such as Mark and Steven.

It is interesting to note in this regard Dell's symbolic transformation at the end of *Afterlife*. Dell actually becomes more economically disenfranchised, more Mexican, as *Afterlife* approaches its conclusion, distancing him even further from the ranks of gay men for whom *Afterlife* promises "happily ever after." Such a transformation is actually predicted by Dell's white lover Marcus as Marcus attempts to put his affairs in order in the days before his death. Marcus fears that Dell will return to Mexico with his sister Linda after he dies—a literal transformation of Dell back into a Mexican—and he tries to make financial arrangements to prevent such an occurrence. "There's life insurance," Marcus tells Linda while Dell is away from the house. "Maybe you can buy some units. But don't go back to Mexico, all right? And don't let *him*" (p. 58).

Marcus' preparations notwithstanding, Dell makes a symbolic return to his ethnic and class origins anyway, penniless and distinctly ethnic by the end of the novel. Although Dell has managed to go from "gardener's helper" (p. 26) to the owner of his own small landscaping company during his time in the States, he abandons such bourgeois trappings as he prepares to kill Mother Evangeline. Dell gives his one truck to his associate Alfonso Nava in exchange for a loaded gun, thereby continuing his earlier move from respectable citizen to "full-fledged outlaw" (p. 143). In trading his business for a gun, in fact, Dell transforms his ethnic identity as well, abandoning the facade of middle-class respectability for the violence Monette associates with Dell's Latino brothers ("Alfonso Nava had come to L.A. from the killing grounds of Guatemala," Monette writes. "He couldn't have cared less what Dell Espinoza wanted with a gun" [p. 246]).

Dell's trip to Mother Evangeline's church furthers this process of ethnic identification and economic decline. Dell transforms himself from gay yuppie to ethnic working class: "He dressed himself in the green fatigues, the blue work shirt, the red bandanna, the very uniform in which he had arrived at Steven's house. Neatly he folded the clothes he'd borrowed from Sonny, which had made him look like any other West Hollywood clone" (p. 266). Although having previously "lived a notch above his immigrant brothers who had no wheels" (p. 267), the new Dell takes the number 41 bus, "a melting pot on wheels" (p. 269) into which he is readily absorbed. Dell identifies most closely with a "gaunt, exhausted Latina" (p. 268) who reminds him of his Mexican mother, and he asks her to pray for him as he exits the bus. Having spent his only cash on the ride into the city, Dell is reduced/returned to the circumstances of an immigrant—forced to take the bus in a city of cars, landing at Mother Evangeline's church without a cent in his pocket.

Dell's transformation at the end of *Afterlife* serves to shore up his status as working-class, ethnic "other," a position that disqualifies him from the class recovery that an end to AIDS would represent for men such as Mark and Steven. In fact, even though Dell meets with an unhappy ending, his fate does little to disrupt *Afterlife*'s metaphoric resolution of the problems AIDS has posed for certain gay men, since Dell was never really one of the gay men in question in the first place. All the more reason, then, to turn him into an activist. Since Dell has no place in the kind of resolutions that *Afterlife* envisions, he becomes an appropriate character on whom to load the burdens of a long-term struggle, one which has no more relevance to "happily ever after" than do the disenfranchised individuals on the number 41 bus.

In one important way, in fact, Dell enables Mark and Steven's happy ending. Dell's obsession with Mother Evangeline has forced the reader (as well as Steven) to acknowledge that love between men might ultimately prove unworkable with homophobes such as Mother Evangeline actively organized against it. Dell's murder/suicide takes care of these complications, however; by killing Mother Evangeline, Dell manages to eliminate whatever political concerns may have lingered in the reader's mind. With Mother Evangeline dead, the forces of homophobia within *Afterlife* die symbolically as well, assuring the reader that the "happily ever after" ending upon which Steven and Mark are depending is viable after all. In having Dell shoot himself, Monette is able to kill two birds with one stone. The need for further struggle is rendered irrelevant; "the sleepers had all they needed" (p. 278).

"THE SAME AS YOU":
LARRY KRAMER'S THE NORMAL HEART

Although generally regarded as one of the most important participants in the literary response to AIDS in this country, Larry Kramer
is probably even better known for his role in the creation and
development of both the Gay Men's Health Crisis (GMHC) and
ACT UP—as well as for his work as a polemicist throughout the
epidemic.[9] As *The Normal Heart* chronicles (however loosely),
Kramer was one of six men who founded GMHC in 1982, creating
what would eventually become the largest AIDS service organization
in the country. Kramer's AIDS work during the early 1980s proved
highly controversial, not only because of the unpopular stances he
often took on subjects such as gay sex or the need for a direct action
response to the epidemic (stances that tended to work their way into
his many speeches and published writings), but also because many of
his opinions clashed directly with the direction in which GMHC's
board wanted that organization to go.[10] Although the majority of the
board viewed the role of that organization as one of providing services to people with AIDS, Kramer's conception of GMHC's role
was grounded in an understanding of "AIDS politics" that was more
in line with what would eventually guide ACT UP—that a "political" response to AIDS was one that was geared to producing institutional change, especially in the way that government agencies were
responding to the epidemic.[11] Increasingly divided from the rest of
GMHC's leadership, Kramer offered his resignation during an argument in 1983 and found the board unwilling to readmit him later.

Kramer devoted much of his energy following his split with GMHC
to the writing and production of *The Normal Heart*. First produced in
1985, the play recounts the history of the early epidemic in New York
through the story of Ned Weeks, a fictional character modeled after
Kramer, who helps to form an AIDS service organization, finds a
lover, and loses both in a series of sixteen scenes that take place
between July 1981 and May 1984.[12] Extremely conventional in terms
of form, *The Normal Heart*'s plot is also relatively straightforward.
Alarmed by the appearance of a strange and often fatal disease among
his gay male friends and associates, Ned Weeks, a New York City
writer, makes the new epidemic his obsession. Ned helps to found an

AIDS service organization, and he becomes the main mouthpiece for
Emma Brookner, a physician who believes that gay men should take
up celibacy until more can be learned about the epidemic.

Meanwhile, Ned's personal life takes several dramatic turns. Ned
feuds with his brother Ben, whom he accuses of being unable to
accept fully Ned's homosexuality, and he begins a relationship with
Felix Turner, a closeted reporter at the *The New York Times* whom he
meets as part of his campaign to increase media coverage of the
epidemic. (Ned berates Felix for his unwillingness to write anything
more serious than fashion columns, but Felix agrees to a date with
him anyway.) The second half of the play is more tragic: Felix
becomes ill himself, and the board of the AIDS organization,
alarmed at both Ned's confrontational style and his constant harping
on celibacy, removes him from its ranks. Felix dies in the final scene
of the play, but not before he and Ned can be joined in a deathbed
marriage ceremony conducted by Emma and witnessed by Ben.

As my plot summary here should suggest, *The Normal Heart*, like
Afterlife, revolves around a central love story, and Kramer has been
explicit in his writings about the role that love story played in his larger
project. "I wrote it to make people cry: AIDS is the saddest thing I'll
ever have to know," Kramer has indicated of his play:

> I also wrote it to be a love story, in honor of a man I loved who
> died. I wanted people to see on a stage two men who loved each
> other. I wanted people to see them kiss. I wanted people to see
> that gay men in love and gay men suffering and gay men dying
> are just like everyone else.[13]

Of course, Kramer's use of the word "people" here is somewhat
disingenuous. Since most gay men in his audience would have
already realized that "gay men . . . are just like everyone else,"
Kramer's generic reference to "people" clearly refers to heterosexuals. For Kramer, a gay love story was viewed as a strategic way to
tap the sympathies of a heterosexual audience. Presented with the
picture of gay men finding and losing love "just like everyone
else," heterosexuals would presumably be moved to do something
about the epidemic.

Another important aspect of Kramer's politics that manifested
itself in his nonfiction writings was an understanding of the epidemic

grounded in his class position as an economically privileged gay man. Kramer has described the shock felt by himself and many other gay men who had experienced the benefits of class privilege during the 1970s but who watched these benefits collapse when AIDS began to devastate their community—a shock, as Kramer put it, that challenged their faith in the liberal promise of equality and democracy. "I . . . learned, after an earlier life of comparative privileges, what it's like not to have them anymore. I have learned—in a more tangible and visible way than I ever thought or was taught I would encounter in a 'free' and 'democratic' society—how gay people are hated and expendable."[14] Having been part of a sector of the gay community that understood itself in terms of parties and discos rather than a nascent gay liberation movement ("when Gay Pride marches started down Fifth Avenue at the end of June, I was on Fire Island,"[15] he has noted), Kramer and others like him were forced to recognize the tenuous nature of their class position once AIDS presented them with a crisis whose solution was not for sale.

However, just as *Afterlife* "resolves" this crisis of consumption through Mark and Steven's union, *The Normal Heart* provides its own resolution through its depiction of the transformation of Ned's brother Ben. Ben functions as the on-stage representative of the white, middle-class heterosexuals for whom *The Normal Heart* was written—the only heterosexual male in a play filled with dying gay men. As such, he is granted representative powers: on behalf of straight, middle-class America, Ben is afforded the symbolic power to grant or deny gay men such as Ned equal access to the power and privileges of straight men like himself.

The Normal Heart is not a very subtle play, and neither Kramer nor Ned is very subtle about what Ben represents. Ned makes clear to Ben that Ben has more power to end the epidemic than any gay person Ned knows, and on two occasions he chastises Ben (and by extension, heterosexuals in the audience) for failing to use this power. The first instance of this process takes place in Scene 3, which occurs in October 1981. Ned begs Ben to make the law firm in which he is a partner take on the AIDS organization as a pro bono client, but Ben is reluctant to do so, insisting that he will have to let the partners decide as a group.

BEN: I'll put it to them at the next meeting.

NED: When is that?

BEN: When it is!

NED: When is it? Because if you're not going to help, I have to find somebody else.

BEN: You're more than free to do that.

NED: I don't want to do that! I want my big brother's fancy famous big-deal straight law firm to be the first major New York law firm to do *pro bono* work for a gay cause.[16]

As Ned's comments here suggest, the significance of Ben's firm over any other one that he could go to is that it is associated in Ned's mind with powerful heterosexuals. As such, although on a literal level all that the AIDS organization will require of the firm is routine work, on a symbolic level it comes to represent the stranglehold that heterosexuals have on the legal fate of gays in this country. By offering Ned the services of his firm, Ben would have the chance to put the power of the law in the service of a group of gay men, a chance that he promptly declines.

In Scene 6 (May 1982), Ben and Ned argue again, although this time the stakes are noticeably higher. For what is revealed in this later scene is that the real power that Ben and his kind possess is the ability to grant or deny men such as Ned equality with themselves. Having convinced another partner in Ben's firm to do the pro bono work for the AIDS organization, Ned tries to persuade his brother to join the honorary board of the organization, an "honor" that Ben again declines. The two men begin arguing about gay life, and Ben ties his reluctance to support Ned's cause to the seemingly incomprehensible practices of Ned and *his* kind: ". . . guys in leather and chains and whips and black masks" (p. 68), men in dresses, and Ned's pre-AIDS weakness for bathhouse sex. ". . . You guys have a dreadful image problem" (p. 68), Ben concludes, and Ned agrees, indicating that this is exactly why heterosexuals such as Ben need to join the cause. ". . . That's what has to be changed," Ned agrees. "That's why it's so important to have people like you supporting us. You're a respected person. You already have your dignity" (p. 68).

Of course, by "dignity," Ned means human dignity, that which entitles an individual to the rights and privileges that come with full personhood, something that men such as Ned are legally and socially denied. More important, however, Ben's dignity, and by extension his personhood, is also what allows him to be the agent of the denial of this personhood to gay men—a process which occurs in society at large, but one which Ben (the representative of heterosexuals) enacts symbolically by refusing to lend his name (the symbol of his personhood) to Ned's honorary board. As Ned makes clear, however, the inability of straight men to see gay men as full persons has very real consequences, as the AIDS epidemic has made painfully clear:

BEN: My agreeing you were born just like I was born is not going to help save your dying friends.

NED: Funny—that's exactly what I think will help save my dying friends. (p. 70)

Ultimately, Ned shows his hand, revealing during the course of his fight with Ben what gay men really want, and what the political struggle that Kramer champions at the end of his play is really all about—not an eradication of the legal, social, and economic privileges that men such as Ben possess, but an extension of these privileges to gay men as well.[17] Ned's project in Scene 6 is ostensibly one of getting Ben to join his board, but it also is one of trying to get Ben to admit that gay men are equal to straight men like himself, an admission that is the crucial step in institutionalizing such a position of equality. At this point in the play, however, Ben is incapable of changing his mind. "You've got to say it. I'm the same as you. Just say it. Say it!" Ned insists, to which Ben can only reply, "No, you're not. I can't say it" (p. 70). Ned is devastated by Ben's refusal and severs his ties with his brother (a split that is not healed until Ben shows up unexpectedly at Ned and Felix's marriage ceremony). ". . . You still think I'm sick," Ned cries out in the lines that end the scene, "and I simply cannot allow that any longer. I will not speak to you again until you accept me as your equal. Your healthy equal. Your brother!" (p. 71).

As Ned's use of the word "brother" emphasizes, Ben's inability to view Ned as his equal is particularly striking because Ben and Ned are in fact brothers, as biologically close as two men can be.

Moreover, because of Ben's investments on his behalf, Ned has a similar class position as that of his older brother. Nonetheless, what Ben and *his* kind also possess is the ability to deny even affluent, white gay men a viable position in the dominant classes, rather than the more tenuous one that certain gay men were able to orchestrate before AIDS, but which fell apart once AIDS undermined their ability to pass, identifying them as a class apart—the men in the "black masks" whom Ben so despises. Recognizing the social and political changes that need to take place before this repositioning can occur, Kramer champions political struggle at the end of his play, as Ned picks up the activist torch once more.[18]

Kramer's pragmatism notwithstanding, *The Normal Heart* engages in its own bit of wishful thinking in its final scene. For although Ned loses one of the things he has always wanted—a lover—at the end of the play, he gains the approval of his brother. Through his surprise appearance at Ned and Felix's "wedding," and his embrace of Ned in the very last second of the play, Ben signifies both a recognition of gay relationships as equal to straight ones and an acknowledgment that Ned is in fact his equal. As such, Ben's transformation at the end of *The Normal Heart* acts as a lesson for the heterosexuals who are the play's intended audience. As with Ben, these audience members are challenged to recognize—and thereby grant—gay men's equality to heterosexuals like themselves. *The Normal Heart* may call for change, and it may recognize that struggle will be necessary to bring this change about, but the kinds of change it advocates are of a relatively unchallenging liberal variety—not the eradication of the privileges enjoyed by men such as Ben, but rather, the extension of these privileges to a group of men who are "the same" as him in every way but one.

UNRECIPROCATED GESTURES: SARAH SCHULMAN'S PEOPLE IN TROUBLE

Sarah Schulman's 1990 novel *People in Trouble* has a lot in common with *Afterlife* and *The Normal Heart:* major characters who are AIDS activists, a love story that is central to the narrative, a nonexperimental structure and style, and an author who was involved with activist politics. At the same time, *People in Trouble* can also be understood as a critique of the project that has been the central focus of this chapter so far—that of rectifying the class dislocation that AIDS produced among middle-class gay men. In Chapter 1, I argued that this class dislocation drove an unlikely group of gay men into grassroots activism for the first time and caused ACT UP to be organized, in part, around the priorities and styles that these men brought with them. Likewise, Chapter 2 has so far considered some of the ways in which two authors attempted to provide an imaginative solution to this class dislocation in their writings.

People in Trouble, by contrast, adopts an entirely different approach to the question of how to address the divisions that AIDS produced between middle-class gay men and their heterosexual counterparts. Although dealing with the same topics that concern Monette and Kramer (albeit via a lesbian protagonist), Schulman offers a critique of a response to AIDS that is grounded in the idea of securing for gay men the same kinds of privileges that straight men possess. This is by no means a separatist project, for Schulman views the gay men who were drawn to ACT UP as integral participants in the political response that she envisions. Nonetheless, Schulman combines an identity politics with a Marxist one in *People in Trouble,* arguing that the privileges that straight men possess must be eradicated, rather than extended to gay men.

In order to understand the critique that structures *People in Trouble,* it is important to have at least some understanding of Schulman's experiences as a lesbian writer, a lesbian activist, and a lesbian in ACT UP. As I discussed in Chapter 1, the political backgrounds of most of the women in ACT UP were considerably different from the men who made up the majority of members, and Schulman, who joined ACT UP in 1987, was no exception to this pattern.[19] Although most of the men in ACT UP eventually became aware of the need to create a movement that would benefit groups besides themselves, many of them came to ACT UP without any previous political experience at all, jolted by the realization that the tenuous position they had crafted for themselves within the dominant classes had been severely jeopardized by the advent of AIDS.[20] As I noted earlier, many of these men did develop an expanded critique of social inequalities while members of ACT UP. But whether they approved of their own class privilege or not, the reality for many gay white men was that their experience of the epidemic—and of inequality in general—was extremely different from that of other disenfranchised groups.

Women, on the other hand, tended to come to ACT UP from a very different perspective. For one thing, since few of these women were sick with HIV themselves, most came to that organization as part of larger personal histories of activist involvement in the feminist and antiwar movements and other leftist and progressive causes, meaning that the women in the group tended to have more political experience than the men and were often already extremely critical of existing social inequalities. Second, although most of these women were, similar to the male activists, middle-class professionals, as women they harbored no illusions that a movement dedicated to ending AIDS could address the inequalities faced by women in the same way that it could address those faced by middle-class gay men.

Openly lesbian writers such as Schulman also have a different relationship to the literary marketplace from that of their gay male (and especially white gay male) counterparts. The author of six novels and a collection of essays, Schulman is one of the most prominent lesbians writing today. Her publication by E.P. Dutton places her in the ranks of but a handful of openly lesbian authors of books with lesbian content who have found mainstream publishers, and her books are widely reviewed in mainstream publications.[21] Nonetheless, Schulman has nothing to match the mainstream awards and recognition that many gay male writers have received (e.g., Paul Monette's National Book Award for *Becoming a Man*). Schulman has commented on this level of institutional discrimination herself. "By 1992 I discovered that I was in a ghetto as a lesbian novelist," she notes in her essay "My Life as an American Artist":

> My fifth novel *Empathy* was published. I got reviewed in *Entertainment Weekly* but still could not get one straight bookstore in New York City to let me read there except during Gay Pride Month. The best-selling books by lesbian writers had no lesbian content. When that content was introduced, the books plummeted in the esteem of critics, book buyers, and the general public.[22]

This is not to say that Schulman's experiences as a lesbian writer and a lesbian activist *prevented* her from adopting the perspectives of certain male activists, but rather that these experiences were instrumental in shaping the critique that is at the bottom of *People in Trouble.*

People in Trouble is a highly polemical novel, and Schulman's critique encompasses a number of topics. Two components of this critique are of particular interest, however, because they are directly related to the project that structured ACT UP, *Afterlife,* and *The Normal Heart*—that of responding to the class dislocation that AIDS produced among middle-class gay men. On the one hand, Schulman provides a blistering indictment in *People in Trouble* of the homophobia of heterosexuals, and especially heterosexual men; on the other hand, she offers a critique of the class styles and political inexperience of the middle-class gay men who were drawn to ACT UP—a combination, as we have seen, that severely limited the reach of that organization early in its history.

The relationship of Schulman's (or any) critique of ACT UP to the question of a middle-class gay male experience of AIDS should be clear by now. What I want to argue in the following pages, however, is that for all its apparent focus on another entirely separate target, Schulman's critique of *heterosexual* men impinges just as strongly on the experiences of gay men as does her focus on AIDS activism itself. I begin my analysis by looking at the elaborate machinery that Schulman employs to launch her critique of the homophobia of heterosexuals. Having outlined the parameters of this critique, I then turn my attention to its surprising relevance to a middle-class *gay* male experience of the epidemic.

Schulman makes use of two intersecting stories in *People in Trouble* in order to explore the issues mentioned above. First and foremost, *People in Trouble* tells the story of a love triangle involving Molly, a lesbian AIDS activist; Kate, a married visual artist who becomes Molly's lover; and Peter, a theatrical lighting designer and Kate's husband. Simultaneously, the novel chronicles the rise of Justice, an AIDS activist organization modeled loosely after ACT UP/ New York. As Molly and Peter struggle for Kate's time and attention, Kate increasingly views her artwork as an inadequate response to the ravages of AIDS and homelessness in New York, and she eventually joins Molly as a member of Justice. *People in Trouble* concludes somewhat ambivalently, however: Molly leaves Kate, frustrated over Kate's continued interest in Peter; Kate leaves Peter; Peter takes a new lover; and Kate abandons her activism in order to do artwork in Europe.

People in Trouble's critique of what Schulman herself termed the "neglect and abandonment of gay people"[23] by heterosexuals is performed along two lines: a realistic portrayal of both Kate's bungled attempts to juggle her two relationships and Peter's reaction to her affair, and a satiric depiction of the real estate magnate Ronald Horne, a character based loosely on Donald Trump. Schulman's treatment of Kate is the most subtle and complicated component of this critique because even as Kate continually manages to fail Molly, she travels a considerable distance while lovers with her insofar as lesbian and gay issues are concerned. Kate becomes sexually involved with a woman, makes lesbian and gay friends, joins an AIDS activist organization, and even begins to cross-dress as a man. Likewise, she distances herself so considerably from Peter's attitudes that she finds it necessary to leave him by the end of the novel. But despite all of this personal development, Kate's homophobia remains so ingrained that it ultimately destroys her relationship with Molly.

Essential to any project of being "accusatory to straight people for their abandonment" of gay people is of course a detailed discussion of homophobia, and the problems that plague Molly and Kate's relationship allow Schulman to demonstrate the impact of homophobia on individual lives. Kate's unresolved homophobia—her refusal to identify as a lesbian, or even with the lesbian community, and her terror of lessening her ties with heterosexual men—overshadows her relationship with Molly at every moment and contributes significantly to that relationship's ultimate collapse. Even a year into the relationship, Kate feels the need to rationalize her involvement with a woman. "Having a girlfriend makes sex better with your man,"[24] she tells herself while walking home from Molly's one evening, and after Molly gives her a tour of lesbian bars and a gay porno shop, Kate insists that "I like cock," even while acknowledging to Molly that she would never say "I like pussy" to Peter (p. 85).

Kate's running into her married friend Susan while on the bar tour with Molly constitutes an especially suggestive example of how her fear of homosexuality and her identification with her husband undermine the personal changes she appears to have made. Even in the safe environment of a lesbian bar, Kate fails to introduce Molly to Susan, continuing a pattern by which she had refused to see Molly under any circumstances that would force Peter to recognize how much time the two women spend together. Schulman writes, "She could feel Molly standing next to her but Kate just didn't want to introduce them. She felt pressured" (p. 81). Kate, in fact, overcompensates for the run-in by training her thoughts on both her own husband and Susan's husband Dan. For one thing, Kate identifies Susan to Molly in terms of Susan's husband: "That woman, I know her. That's Susan Hoffman. Her husband is a sculptor" (p. 81). And she responds to her uneasiness at seeing Susan in the bar by focusing the conversation on Peter and Dan, even as Susan shows no interest in hearing about Peter and makes a veiled reference to her own lesbian lover:

> "Isn't this strange?" Kate said. "All these women dressed up like this. I mean, it's nice."
>
> "Yeah," Susan said. "Nice."

Then Kate noticed that Susan was dressed up too.

> "How's Dan?"
>
> "Fine."
>
> "Pete's fine too."
>
> "That's good. Oh, there's my friend. See you later."
>
> "Will I see you and Dan at Jack's party on Saturday night?"
>
> "Yeah, we'll be there."
>
> "So will me and Pete."
>
> "See you then."
>
> "See you." (p. 81)

Molly uses the incident to attack Kate's heterosexist view of the world, but to little avail. When Kate insists that Susan could not be a lesbian because "I know her husband," Molly retorts, "You think you're the only closeted married woman in New York City?" To which Kate replies, "I am not closeted" (p. 82).

Kate's attempts throughout *People in Trouble* to protect Peter from her homosexuality (or at least her sexual experimentation) constitute an important component of a larger process in which dominant and subordinate constituencies are repeatedly mistaken by characters in the novel. Within Kate's logic, Peter becomes the victim (a role he adopts readily, as we shall see), and homosexuality, the oppressing force. Rather than attempting to protect Molly from homophobia (e.g., Peter's), Kate goes out of her way to protect Peter from homosexuality (e.g., her affair), a project that becomes all the more apparent to Molly when she "cheats" on Kate with a lesbian named Sam. Walking home from an activist meeting with Molly, Sam "put her arm around Molly and protected her from men on the street who said stupid insulting things to them all the way to Sam's house" (p. 179). Having finally been "protected" by her lover, Molly recognizes Kate's misplaced priorities.

Although Schulman's feelings about Kate remain somewhat ambivalent, her antipathy toward Peter is less mistakable. As Schulman indicated in an interview in *The Women's Review of Books*, however, she deliberately went out of her way while writing *People in Trouble* to avoid turning Peter into a monster. "I had to make Peter be better than I really believed him to be," she explained. "It's the only time in my life that I've ever lied about a character. What I did to 'humanize' him was make him be me. I put all of my personal stuff into him. I gave him the most attention, and so he's the most developed character."[25] Schulman's use of three separate narrative perspectives in her novel also assists in making Peter an occasionally empathetic character. Although *People in Trouble* is narrated from the third person throughout, the narration in each chapter is filtered through either Kate's, Molly's, or Peter's point of view through the use of free indirect discourse. Since most of Peter's activities occur in chapters narrated from his perspective, his own inability to recognize the shortcomings of his actions means that nothing exists in the narration of these chapters to explicitly challenge his world view, so that any detection of Schulman's critique requires reading between the lines. (By contrast, in scenes in which Molly's perspective is dominant, Peter generally gets slammed hard.)

Peter's shortcomings fall into three areas: his feelings of superiority to people who are different from himself (and his need to continually remind himself of this superiority); his tendency to view himself as the victim in his relationship with people who are normally viewed as subordinate to heterosexual men (such as gays); and his unwillingness to take action in the face of large-scale social problems. Schulman begins her implicit critique of Peter early in the novel, during a scene in which he goes out for one of his frequent jogs. Peter notices that "all along the route someone had spray-painted the word *Justice* inside stencils of pink triangles" (p. 27). Unfamiliar with the AIDS activist organization that his wife will soon join, Peter misidentifies "Justice," as "just another rock band," but this process of misidentification also points to Peter's unfamiliarity with what "justice" might mean as a philosophical concept as well, an unfamiliarity that will manifest itself throughout the novel. Peter stops in a restaurant for an iced tea, and he reacts strongly to a group of gay men at a nearby table. "Peter noticed that his own chest was twice the size of theirs" (p. 29), Schulman writes, an irrelevant observation on his part, no doubt, but one which provides an initial instance of his need to remind himself of his imagined superiority to gay men.

This line of logic continues when Peter notices an AIDS funeral entering the church across the street. Even while focusing on the mourners, Peter is able to position himself as the victimized party in his relationship with homosexuals, as well as, through a strange twist of logic, a casualty of the epidemic. "Ever since Kate had begun her gay affair," Schulman narrates from Peter's perspective, "Peter had been slapped in the face by homosexuality practically every day. How ironic that her affair had coincided with this AIDS thing" (p. 31). Upon leaving the restaurant, Peter does decide that "he wanted to be around gay people more" but his decision has nothing to do with a desire to get to know gay people better. Rather, in the same way that Kate justifies sex with Molly as a way to improve her relationship with Peter, Peter envisions that being "around gay people more" will help bring him and Kate "closer together" (p. 32).

Peter's warped perspective becomes particularly apparent during Justice's invasion of Ronald Horne's "Castle," a luxury hotel with a colonial theme. Watching the television news at a bar, Peter reacts strongly when the anchorman announces a story on AIDS: " 'Oooh, I'm so sick of AIDS,' Peter groaned. He couldn't help himself" (p. 123). Peter's announcement here is loaded with irony, of course: although it is people with AIDS who are the ones who are actually "sick of AIDS," Peter is only able to view the epidemic as it affects him as a heterosexual man.[26] Likewise, Peter's announcement to his lover Shelley that he needs "a break" (p. 170) from homosexuality positions him once again as the victim of homosexuals and homosexuality, masking the ways in which homosexuals are victimized by homophobes like himself.

Peter's ability to view himself as oppressed finds its greatest manifestation during a scene in which he comes across a group of homeless and poor people waiting to enter a soup kitchen (the scene is again narrated from Peter's perspective, allowing him to escape a thorough trouncing). "When he started looking at these people," Schulman reports, "Peter felt a deep, deep compassion. It drew him closer to them, this sense of injustice that they had been treated so badly" (p. 135). Feeling mistreated at the hands of his wife, Peter has the audacity to identify with the oppression of the homeless, as Schulman's use of the ambiguous "they" (meaning both "the homeless" and "Peter and the homeless") signifies. Such a process of identification, of course, serves to mask (at least in his mind) the amount of social and economic power Peter has in relation to those people who have gathered for the meal. Even if Peter were oppressed (which Schulman makes clear he is not), such a move fails to recognizes the differences that exist in various forms of oppression, differences that create opportunities for one oppressed class of people to work on behalf of another.

As Schulman makes clear, however, Peter's undeserved gesture of identification goes only so far. Although Peter might be able to muster up some compassion for the homeless and hungry, he is ultimately unwilling to do anything to improve their situation:

How can you relieve suffering for even one moment? he thought. *Here we are, the homeless, the old, the artists. The sadness is so overwhelming I can't imagine what to do. Nothing in my life has prepared me for this.* (p. 137)

Here, Peter says the magic words. For it is the unwillingness of people such as Peter to take action in the face of suffering (except, perhaps, to imagine that they are suffering too) that comes under the strongest attack in *People in Trouble.* "We are a people in trouble" the Justice activist James announces in the penultimate paragraph of the novel. "We do not act" (p. 228), a position that is also articulated earlier in the novel when Molly reminds Kate that "Here in New York City there are people who take action and people who do nothing. Doing nothing is a position. It means giving approval without having to actively say so" (p. 165).

Ronald Horne is the other straight white male with a major role in *People in Trouble,* and his presence serves to represent the societal consequences of Peter's attitudes and behaviors—the way in which, as Schulman put it, "how people feel about us [gays and lesbians] . . . translates into public policy."[27] Horne is a larger-than-life version of Peter, one who fails to disguise his homophobia and disdain for the poor with liberal platitudes and self-justification and who carries Peter's prejudices to their logical consequences. Peter verbalizes his contempt for gay men; Horne attempts to evict them from the apartment complexes he has purchased. Peter wants AIDS out of his life; mayoral candidate Horne proposes quarantining PWAs on barges in the harbor. Horne's presence in New York City is inescapable (he continually buys up property such as cinemas and the public library), but references to Horne generally appear in the scenes that are narrated from Peter's perspective, again suggesting the affinities between the two men. Peter notices Horne more than any other character does because Horne is the character who is most like him.

Although Schulman's critique of people such as Kate, Horne, and especially Peter should be evident at this point, the connection of this critique to the AIDS-related experiences of financially secure gay men is less obvious. Although Schulman is clearly able to criticize the behavior of heterosexuals through Peter and Kate, I would argue that the two of them also act as a negative object lesson for middle-class gay men in general, and for the politically inexperienced gay men who joined the early ACT UP in particular. This is not because Peter and Kate are homophobic. Rather, it is because they are willing to abandon groups of people who are different from themselves, either explicitly (as when Peter views himself as the oppressed party in his relationship with gays or when Kate refuses to identify as a lesbian) or through neglect (as when Peter determines that there is nothing he can do to assist the homeless with whom he so inappropriately identifies).

Peter's unwillingness to do anything to benefit people who are different from himself and his smug sense of superiority to others provide examples of a politics that falls far short of Schulman's personal understanding of a radical politics. As Schulman indicated in my interview with her, a "radical" politics is one in which "you take your place in a larger movement for freedom for everybody. That you're not just there for yourself." "It's how you see yourself in relation to other people," she added. "If you see yourself as one with other people, or you think that you're better." By representing the consequences for gay people when heterosexuals fail to adopt such a politics, Peter's behavior simultaneously manages to suggest the similar consequences that occur when gay people fail to make connections with people who are different from *them*selves (women, people of color, injection drug users, the homeless). Moreover, Peter and Kate's unwillingness to recognize power differentials between themselves and other groups of people represents an implicit call for middle-class gay men to recognize that, even as they themselves are suffering from a form of oppression with deadly consequences, and are thus disempowered to a great extent, they simultaneously hold the power to do something about the kinds of oppression being experienced by other groups. In other words, by offering them a character who only thinks in terms of his own needs, Schulman challenges her readers to ask themselves if they really wish to act in the same way.

Significantly enough, this was exactly the problem that Schulman witnessed occurring in the early ACT UP—a problem that was not entirely unexpected for a group of people without an extensive history in movement politics, but which in many ways hampered the early work of the group. "It was not clear how radical an organization [ACT UP] was going to be from the beginning," Schulman explained:

because the vast majority of men in ACT UP had never been politically active before. That is to say, they had never advocated on behalf of anyone before. So, for the women, for the most part, and the handful of gay men who had political backgrounds—who had been in the feminist movement for ten years previous, or whatever—it was frustrating in many ways. . . . So initially I wanted to sort of chide them for not being radical enough, or not being dramatic enough.[28]

What is particularly significant about Schulman's challenge to her readers, however, is that it manages to comment upon not only the workings of ACT UP, but also the entire project of rectifying the class dislocations that AIDS produced among middle-class gay men. As we have already seen, this project can go in one of two directions. On the one hand, it can take a narrow focus—one geared toward trying to extend (or more accurately reextend) to white, middle-class gay men many of the privileges of their heterosexual counterparts. On the other hand, it can take a broader focus—one which attempts to address the power imbalance that exists between gay and straight men by eradicating the privileges the latter hold, not by winning for gay men the same set of privileges. The reason why this second approach represents a "broader" (or to use Schulman's term more "radical") politics, however, is because its end result would be to improve the social and political status of all oppressed groups, not just gay men. In other words, it is a coalition politics, not just a gay one. By demonstrating the murderous consequences that straight male privilege and self-absorption have had for *gay men themselves,* then, Schulman challenges the notion that the best way of addressing the class dislocation gay men have experienced is to work toward winning for gay men the exact same set of privileges.

Although Peter's warped perspectives provide an indirect means through which Schulman is able to challenge a political project— and a political movement—based strictly on the needs of its own participants, she addresses this problem head-on in other places in the novel as well. At times, for instance, Schulman comments explicitly on the class styles that middle-class gay men brought with them upon joining a grassroots movement for the first time. When the character Scott makes announcements at the beginning of a Justice meeting, for instance, Schulman expresses her ambivalence

about the nature of an activist movement organized around an unexpected loss of class privilege. "Scott began the meeting with a list
of announcements," Schulman narrates:

> As he read from the notes he played unconsciously with his
> pony-tail, twisting the hair around the forefinger of his right
> hand. He had a combined air of enthusiasm and serious deter-
> mination: like a middle-class boy who one day discovered
> injustice and then proceeded to do something about it with both
> sincere conviction and class arrogance about getting things
> done his way. (p. 116)

Later in the same scene, Schulman takes a jab at a character who
questions the viability of the demonstration at the Horne Castle: his
imagination limited by "a lot of discretionary income," the young
man wonders how the hundreds of people attending the Justice meeting will ever be able to find cabs (p. 119). Finally, in describing a
later Justice meeting, Schulman is quite clear about the class backgrounds of most of the men in the room: "There were distinguished
homosexuals with white-boy jobs, who had forgotten that they were
queer until AIDS came along and everyone else reminded them"
(p. 158).

Schulman also critiques a "me-first" politics through her inclusion of a scene in which the character James explains his personal
project of trying to transform AIDS from "an overwhelming personal void into a group effort, to try to help others avoid the same
fate" (p. 147). Based on his readings about "the Holocaust, about
Hiroshima, slavery, and apartheid" (p. 147), James comes to the
conclusion that "when a person faces death . . . especially a deliberate, uncalled-for and avoidable death, they only seem to have two
reactions. *Why me?* and *I don't want to die*" (p. 147). Although
recognizing the difficulty of going beyond such thinking (James
ultimately adopts such a perspective himself), Schulman uses this
scene to challenge her readers to think of an AIDS movement as
potentially benefiting others besides themselves.

Schulman's most imaginative way of addressing the problem of
political nearsightedness within ACT UP, however, consists of providing a positive example of what a movement such as ACT UP might
become—her depiction of a fanciful, utopian Justice action called

"Credit Card Day." Having collected the credit cards of people with AIDS who are close to death or have recently died, Justice organizes a gigantic shopping spree for the poor of New York. Groceries for the homeless, fur coats for residents of a women's shelter, "electrical and construction supplies for the Lower East Side squatters," and "one-way tickets" for people wanting to return to "Jamaica, Puerto Rico, and Miami Beach" (p. 208) are paid for with the credit cards, under the assumption that the owners of the cards are close enough to death that they will never have to pay for the charges themselves.

Credit Card Day is a moment of multiple significances for *People in Trouble,* not the least of which is that it held a personal importance to Schulman herself. As both an activist and a writer, Schulman was deeply concerned with making connections between AIDS and home-lessness. Schulman became active with the Housing Committee in ACT UP, and in 1988, she published an article in the *Nation* titled "Thousands May Die in the Streets: AIDS and the Homeless."[29] Committed to making connections between these issues herself, then, Schulman included Credit Card Day in her novel, as, in part, a way of pushing ACT UP to continue to make similar connections.

Credit Card Day functions to bring together and ultimately resolve a number of the issues that have assumed importance in *People in Trouble.* For one thing, by representing a response (however fanciful) to the problem of homelessness, Credit Card Day stands in sharp contrast to Peter's inability to "imagine what to do" (p. 137) upon witnessing the homeless in the soup kitchen. Peter philosophizes; Justice acts. Second, and just as significantly, Credit Card Day constitutes an imagined moment in which affluent gay men dying from AIDS are able to look beyond their own suffering (which Schulman acknowl-edges as being tremendously real) and ask themselves in what ways they still retain certain levels of social and economic privilege, and how that privilege might be mobilized on behalf of other disenfran-chised populations. What the men who donate their credit cards to Justice have, of course, is financial clout—the ability to get Master-Card and Visa to lend them money. Recognizing that there is nothing left for them to buy that could possibly meet their needs, however, these men lend their financial power to homeless people, whose needs *can* be met through the working of the market. Such a response stands in sharp contrast to that of Peter, who, imagining himself to be one of the oppressed, decides that he has no obligation to assist others. As such, Credit Card Day constitutes a moment in which differentials of power among oppressed groups are accounted for and acted upon and the imagined linkages that Peter believes he is forging with disenfranchised groups (linkages that always end up reproducing a situation of inequality) are replaced with real ones.

Credit Card Day also serves to undermine everyday processes of commodification and consumption—processes which I have already argued have been central to the thinking and activism surrounding the epidemic, and which are exemplified in *People in Trouble* by the acquisitive dealings of Horne. Horne's privatization campaign involves taking things that are normally not viewed as commodities (the New York harbor, the New York Public Library), and transforming them into private property that can be bought and sold on the market. What Credit Card Day manages to do, however, is to reverse this process. Since the goods the Justice activists purchase will never be paid for, they are (at least on a symbolic level) stripped of their value (no money will go to their producers) and returned to the status of strictly useful things—food and clothing that the homeless will put to immediate use.

Such a process stands in sharp contrast to consumption as the Horne family practices it, as is illustrated by a picture on the cover of *New York* magazine depicting the family seated around a "bountiful dinner table," "huge portions" of food covering the men's plates (p. 30). As with Horne, the gay men who donate their charge cards to Credit Card Day possess a good deal of disposable income, and on one level, they, similar to Horne, end up purchasing much more than they will ever be able to use. The twist, of course, is that the purchases will go to the homeless: stumped by the contradiction of having the ability to purchase anything they want, but being unable to buy the one thing they really need, the charge card donors in effect transfer their purchasing power to a group of people who have none. By allowing them to distance their consumption practices from those of the Hornes, then, Credit Card Day creates a moment when affluent gay men choose to act like something besides their heterosexual counterparts. Moreover, these men do so knowing that the homeless will never be able to do anything to help them in return. This, however, is entirely Schulman's point. Of such seemingly unreciprocated gestures, she suggests, are real coalitions made.

PART TWO:
LOVE AND POLITICS

Chapter 3

Strange Bedfellows:
Writing Love and Politics
in *Angels in America*
and *The Normal Heart*

Don't come from anger, come from love.[1]

—Tim in *Afterlife*

One of the results of the recent attempt among theater scholars to distinguish between "first" and "second generation" AIDS plays has been that important similarities between texts relegated to opposing ends of this great divide have been rendered increasingly invisible.[2] Two of the most celebrated AIDS plays written in the United States— Tony Kushner's *Angels in America* (1993) and Larry Kramer's *The Normal Heart* (1985)—have rarely been viewed in terms of what they have in common, in large part because of the years that separated their writing.[3] Nonetheless, both plays contain a remarkable number of similarities, ones which can be traced to the dual commitments of their respective authors: a personal commitment to political struggle, especially in relation to AIDS (both writers were AIDS activists), and an artistic commitment to reaching out to as wide and mainstream an audience as possible.[4] Kramer and Kushner address this first commitment through an explicit treatment of AIDS politics in their plays: both *Angels in America* and *The Normal Heart* raise audience consciousness as to the complicity of government players in the spread of the epidemic, as well as to the political struggles that will be necessary if the epidemic is to end. Political struggle is not a particularly popular topic, however, and what has simultaneously allowed these plays to reach broad audiences is their organization around one or more love stories, a dominant theatrical convention that can render a story about homosexuals and AIDS palatable—even recognizable—to mainstream audiences.

These two plot lines—love and politics—make strange bedfellows, however.[5] Whereas the love story in literature focuses on private relations, politics is generally about public struggle. Whereas a focus on love tends to privilege the individual and the couple, a focus on politics—and especially AIDS politics—generally privileges *collective* forms of action.[6] Most important, in imaginative literature about AIDS at least, love and politics possess an opposing relation to the question of narrative closure. On the one hand, the love plot requires narrative closure: once the "lack" that drives the plot has been satisfied through the union of the lovers, complications are resolved, "happily ever after" is achieved, and the need for further narrative is over.[7] Closure is important even in the case of a tragic love story— even if the love relationship ends unhappily, complications are resolved by the end of the text. In other words, once a protagonist has either succeeded or failed in finding love, a drama can end, for there is nothing else about this character's story that the audience need know.

A plot having to do with political struggle around AIDS, on the other hand, must necessarily eschew narrative closure. Although the love plot in a drama might be resolvable (either tragically or comically) within the time frame the play affords, unless the play contains scenes that occur in the future, the struggle against AIDS cannot be. AIDS—and the fight to end it—will continue long into the future, and if a play is to advocate the kinds of political struggles that could end the epidemic, then the closure upon which the love plot depends must be abandoned in favor of a more open ending ("the struggle continues" instead of "happily ever after").[8] What all of this means, then, is that despite their attempts to write both love and politics into their plays, dramatists such as Kramer and Kushner must eventually endorse one of these plot lines over the other.[9]

Angels in America and *The Normal Heart* make strange bedfellows in themselves. Few commentators have drawn connections between the two plays, and Kushner's play has tended to draw considerably more praise than Kramer's, especially among gay commentators.[10]

By viewing these two plays in relationship to their respective negotiations of love and politics, however, we can begin to map out their remarkable similarities.

THE NORMAL HEART

Ever since its first New York production in 1985, *The Normal Heart* has received a tremendous amount of critical attention (both scholarly and popular), a combined effect of a number of factors: the play's status as one of the first important cultural responses to AIDS, the previous prominence of its author, its appeal to gay and straight audiences alike, its original New York run of over a year, and its subsequent translation and production around the world.[11] As any survey of this critical response would indicate, however, commentators have been extremely divided over the politics of Kramer's play. On the one hand, a number of commentators have viewed *The Normal Heart* as a brilliant intervention into mid-1980s AIDS politics, given what they have understood to be its relentless lashing out at government and media inaction, its humanizing depiction of gay men in general and PWAs in specific, its critique of homophobia and heterosexism, and its attempt to inspire an activist response within the gay community.[12] At the same time, other commentators have viewed Kramer's play as excessively melodramatic, reactionary in both content and form, hypocritical (at best) in its views on sex, and/or a self-glorifying and gross distortion of Kramer's own involvement with the Gay Men's Health Crisis (GMHC).[13]

As the following analysis of *The Normal Heart* will reveal, a number of the arguments in favor of and opposed to Kramer's play possess critical merit.[14] Given the amount of criticism that already exists on *The Normal Heart,* however, it is not my intention to add unnecessarily to debates that have been going on for over a decade now. What I do want to do in this section, however, is consider *The Normal Heart* from a different perspective, one which explains many of Kramer's authorial decisions in terms of his somewhat failed attempt to negotiate the love/politics binarism that I sketched out in the introduction to this chapter.

My approach here represents a significant departure from previous critical approaches to the play, for many commentators (including

Kramer himself) have viewed the twists and turns of *The Normal Heart* as Kramer's attempt to tell a particular kind of story about the early years of AIDS or to push a particular polemic concerning activism or sex. Such an approach is not entirely without merit, but in the case of *The Normal Heart,* it has tended to produce an excessively heated response, especially among the play's detractors. A number of the essays cited above, for instance, criticize *The Normal Heart* for its distortion of the facts, as though in writing his play, Kramer set out to lie about the early years of the epidemic as a means of preserving his place in the history books.[15] Similarly, David Bergman has expressed confusion over the fact that a number of the more reactionary turns in *The Normal Heart* seem to contradict the politics expressed in Kramer's nonfiction writings.[16] In both cases, such thinking implies that Kramer is either a liar or a fool, unable to see the ways in which he is either distorting the past or contradicting himself in writing his play.

What I would like to argue, however, is something different: such contradictions and distortions—in fact, Kramer's entire telling of his story—are influenced not so much by Kramer's political stances on particular issues such as monogamy or the direction of GMHC, but by the politics of form, which requires writers to choose between their love and politics plots. What prevents Kramer from telling the "real" story of his involvement with GMHC, in other words, are the requirements of imaginative literature themselves.

In order to discuss the ways in which Kramer's negotiation of his love and politics plots drives many of the choices he makes for his play, I intend to provide readings for a number of key scenes in *The Normal Heart,* in roughly the order the scenes occur. In a number of instances, my readings will offer explanations for seeming contradictions, incongruities, or gaps in Kramer's text that many critics have attributed to misguided politics or simply sloppy writing. In other instances, I will provide new readings for scenes in the play that have made perfect sense to most readers and viewers, given their assumption that Kramer is simply being faithful to the actual circumstances of his involvement with GMHC. My analysis begins with two questions that, in my reading, can be explained through Kramer's heavy bias toward his love plot for much of the play: (1) Why does Ned take a lover when his political platform revolves heavily around gay men abstaining from sex until more can be learned about the epidemic? (2) Why does Ned get removed from the board of the unnamed AIDS organization?

As mentioned earlier, one of the most frequent reasons why commentators have denounced *The Normal Heart* is because of the sexual politics of the play. Most significant, Ned becomes an active spokesman for Dr. Emma Brookner's recommendation that gay men abstain from having sex until the causes of the new epidemic have been determined, and as the protagonist of the play, as well as a fairly obvious stand-in for Kramer himself, Ned and his proclamations carry considerable weight. Emma presents Ned with his charge as early as Scene 1 of *The Normal Heart:*

> **NED:** And you want me to tell every gay man in New York to stop having sex?
>
> **EMMA:** Who said anything about just New York?
>
> **NED:** You want me to tell every gay man across the country—
>
> **EMMA:** Across the world! That's the only way this disease will stop spreading.
>
> **NED:** Dr. Brookner, isn't that just a tiny bit unrealistic?
>
> **EMMA:** Mr. Weeks, if having sex can kill you, doesn't anybody with half a brain stop fucking?[17]

Despite his initial skepticism, Ned quickly adopts Emma's line of thinking. In fact, although occasionally seeming to temper his "no sex" position with an advocacy of monogamy, Ned tries to get the newly formed AIDS organization to incorporate Emma's guidelines into its flyers, a move that the rest of the board resists. Whereas Mickey, another member of the board, views the creation of an organization brochure as a chance to make an intervention into the scapegoating of the gay community, Ned wants to include in the brochure an essay that notes, among other things, ". . . I am sick of guys moaning that giving up careless sex until this blows over is worse than death . . . I am sick of guys who can only think with their cocks" (p. 57; second ellipsis in original).

Although presented under the guise of "medical authority," Emma's recommendations—and Ned's subscription to them—have strong ideological overtones. For one thing, Emma's "scientific" recommendations align themselves readily with what Ned freely admits is his discomfort with the "promiscuity" aspect of the gay liberation movement. ". . . [A]ll we've created is generations of guys who can't deal with each other as anything but erections" (p. 58), Ned argues at a meeting of the organization, a position echoed in his later claim that ". . . more sex isn't more liberating. And having so much sex makes finding love impossible" (p. 61). More important, Ned's pronouncements have their origins in a similar discomfort with sex that Kramer himself expressed during the early years of AIDS (Ned's comments about "careless sex," for instance, are taken almost word for word from an opinion piece Kramer wrote for the *New York Native* in March 1983).[18]

However, Ned's (and Kramer's) commitment to a politics of celibacy creates one of several massive contradictions within *The Normal Heart*. For at the same time that he attempts to get gay men as a group to stop having sex, Ned becomes involved in a relationship himself. Admittedly, Ned and Felix's relationship is monogamous—even conjugal—in nature, having little to do with the promiscuous sex that Ned most vehemently decries. Nonetheless, Ned's relationship manages to violate the premises of his antisex campaign in several important ways. For one thing, as both Ned and Emma realize, monogamy is no guarantee of protection from infection. ". . . All it takes is one wrong fuck," Ned points out to his skeptical associates at the AIDS organization. "That's not promiscuity—that's bad luck" (p. 101), a concern echoed as Felix considers the possibility that it might have been Ned himself who infected him. Emma, in fact, is outraged at Ned's having entered into a relationship—however monogamous—given his seeming commitment to her antisex campaign. "God damn you!" she replies to the news, a comment that provokes even Ned to reply, "What are we supposed to do—be with nobody ever?" (p. 80). Finally, although Ned and Felix's relationship is ultimately conjugal in nature, the text gives one every reason to believe that the two men end up in bed with each other on the first date, a seeming contradiction to a program of seeking out a marriage-equivalent situation as a protection against the epidemic. Thus, whether one views Ned as adopting a strictly no-sex stance or merely promoting monogamy, Ned's involvement with Felix comes across as hypocritical.

One ready explanation for Ned's violation of his own principles here is that Kramer is using Ned's hypocrisy to demonstrate how unrealistic the expectation is that gay men can simply take up celibacy as a response to AIDS. Since Kramer himself has argued that he attempted in *The Normal Heart* to create as critical a portrait of Ned (and by extension himself) as possible, such a reading would view Ned's waffling on sex-related issues as merely one example of what Kramer felt to be the self-critical nature of his play.[19] What I want to argue here, however, is that Kramer undermines his polemic by incorporating a love story into his play because *The Normal Heart* would fail in its mission of reaching middle-class, heterosexual theatergoers without one. As mentioned earlier, the love story is an excellent vehicle for conveying a challenging political message to mainstream audiences more familiar with dominant theatrical conventions than with calls for political change. By organizing his play around a love story, Kramer prevents *The Normal Heart* from becoming one long polemic, transforming it instead into a satisfying theatrical experience to which mainstream audiences can easily relate.[20]

Kramer's inclusion of a love story in his play seems to have had the desired effect. As Joseph Papp (the artistic director of the Public Theater) wrote in his introduction to the published version of *The Normal Heart:*

> In his moralistic fervor, Larry Kramer is a first cousin to nineteenth-century Ibsen and twentieth-century Odets and other radical writers of the 1930s. Yet, at the heart of *The Normal Heart,* the element that gives this powerful political play its essence, is love—love holding firm under fire, put to the ultimate test, facing and overcoming our greatest fear: death.[21]

Likewise, although William A. Henry III, writing in *Time,* complained that "audience members may feel inclined to tune out during the protracted debate over the direction of gay political movements, and Playwright Kramer belabors his belief that the proper response to AIDS is universal sexual abstinence, at least among gays," he lauded the play for, among other things, "creat[ing] a complex, interesting romance between his surrogate . . . and a New York *Times* fashion reporter."[22] Thus, although a love story might appear to make little sense in a play whose protagonist's project (as well as that of its author) ostensibly revolves around getting gay men to stop having sex, it proves to be an effective—and, I am arguing, necessary—component of a play that is committed to the broader political agenda I have just described. Although Ned might tout a "no sex" message, he has little "choice" but to fall in love.

A second occurrence in *The Normal Heart* that can be read in terms of Kramer's negotiation of love and politics is Ned's removal from the board of the AIDS organization he helped to found. Critics have traditionally read Ned's removal from the board as an entirely unproblematic moment in the play, one requiring no further explanation than Kramer's own rocky departure from GMHC. As I have discussed already, however, the fact that certain events in *The Normal Heart* resemble actual occurrences in Kramer's life by no means guarantees that Kramer has constructed his play to be an accurate historical document. Since numerous important events in Kramer's involvement with GMHC have been either left out or embellished in the play (as many of its detractors were quick to note), it is extremely important that all occurrences in *The Normal Heart*—even those closely aligned with actual historical circumstances—be read as constructed, and that the play as a whole be understood as an imaginative text.

With this in mind, then, I would suggest that Ned's removal from the board of the AIDS organization be read as an important turning point in Kramer's negotiation of the love/politics binarism. Because of the constraints that I described earlier—the love story's drive toward narrative closure, the oppositions that exist between public struggle and private lives, and between collectivity and the individual/couple—Kramer's attempt to fashion Ned as both a lover and an activist cannot succeed indefinitely. As a solution to this problem, then, Ned gets fired from the board. Such a move serves two purposes. First, it allows *The Normal Heart* to position itself definitively on the side of love: fired from the board, Ned no longer has the option of even being an activist, which means that Kramer can devote the remainder of the play to Ned and Felix's relationship—a plot line that is more interesting to audiences anyway.[23] Second,

Ned's removal from the board allows Kramer to favor his love plot without having to denounce activism explicitly, in that Ned's original reason for threatening to leave the board is that he feels the AIDS organization is not activist enough. "... [T]hey've decided they only want to take care of patients," Ned complains to Emma:

> —crisis counseling, support groups, home attendants . . . I know that's important, too. But I thought I was starting with a bunch of Ralph Naders and Green Berets, and the first instant they have to take a stand on a political issue and fight, almost in front of my eyes they turn into a bunch of nurses' aides. (p. 79; second ellipsis in original)

By arranging for Ned to be removed from the board, then, Kramer gets the best of both worlds. On the one hand, such a move allows him to endorse the love plot in his text, an endorsement that is an essential component of his project of writing a conventional tale that mainstream audiences can take to heart. On the other hand, it creates a situation in which Kramer can continue to give lip service to an activist movement that he himself has been extremely committed to at periods in his life. Ned's removal from the board constitutes the exact moment at which this movement is purged from the play, but through a narrative sleight of hand, Kramer is able to embrace love in the service of activism.

A consideration of Kramer's negotiation of his love and politics plots can also help to explain the events that conclude *The Normal Heart*. Although *The Normal Heart*'s love plot receives narrative priority in all the instances I have just described, the play's final scene constitutes an important turning point in which this process is as least partially reversed. Ironically, the play's romance narrative seems to reach full force in this scene: in a move criticized by most of the play's detractors for its bourgeois conventionality, Ned and Felix marry in a ceremony conducted by Emma in Felix's hospital room— an occurrence that, as David Román has argued, "offer[s] the traditional closure of conventional narratives of heterosexual love."[24] The scene then shifts from the sentimental to the maudlin, as Felix dies immediately after the completion of the ceremony.

Without question, Ned and Felix's marriage represents *The Normal Heart*'s final nod to the ideological supremacy of romantic love, and detractors of the play have generally pointed to Felix's death as yet another instance of what they have viewed as the reactionary politics that drive the play. John Clum has argued, for instance, that although *The Normal Heart* gives lip service to romantic relationships between men, Kramer's elimination of Felix promotes an entirely different ideology: gay men must be punished for their past promiscuity, and AIDS has made gay love impossible to find.[25] Likewise, David Román has understood Felix's death as the predictable outcome of Kramer's reliance on a dominant medium (realism) for the depiction of the experiences of a marginalized group (gays). "Realist drama is so imbedded in the prevailing ideology of naturalized heterosexuality in dominant culture," Román argues, "that it offers no representational position for gay men or lesbians which is not marginal or a site of defeat."[26]

Although both of these critics have a point, what I would like to suggest is that as much as it promotes dominant ideologies, Felix's death is even more significant in the way that it allows Kramer to *reverse* the ideological trajectory of his play—albeit at a very late moment. As we have seen, Kramer has the choice in *The Normal Heart* of endorsing either his love or his politics plot, and he throws in his lot with the former from as early as Scene 2 in the play (when Ned and Felix meet). By killing off Felix, however, Kramer puts an end to the narrative dominance of his love plot, thereby creating both a literal space in which Ned can become an activist again and an ideological space in which the play can begin to recover its support for an activist agenda.

Several occurrences in the last scene of *The Normal Heart* point to the play's reendorsement of an activist politics. In the first place, it is important to remember that of the two men who make up *The Normal Heart*'s central relationship, Ned (the activist) is the one who remains alive at the end of the play, while Felix (who preferred a more domestic role) is dead. Second, the play offers several suggestions that Ned's activist work is about to resume following the hiatus that occurred when he was removed from the board of the AIDS organization. Felix, on his deathbed, asks Ned to ". . . [p]lease learn to fight again" (p. 121), and Ned informs Felix that he has in fact already begun the process by attempting to attend a meeting of gay leaders to which he was not invited. Felix's actual death, however, is what ultimately reminds Ned that activism is the only way that the lives of people such as Felix might be saved. "Why didn't I fight harder!" he asks his brother, who has made an unexpected appearance for the wedding. "Why didn't I picket the White House, all by myself if nobody would come. Or go on a hunger strike" (p. 122). Even without an organization to back him up, Ned realizes, some political gesture might have been made.

What is most significant about Felix's death, however, is that although occurring very near to the end of the play, it is not in fact what ends it. Even though a tragic love story—with its attendant catharsis—can lend itself to closure as readily as a comic one, Kramer resists ending his play with Felix's death. Instead, he extends his text beyond the confines of the love story, gesturing to the political struggle that must and will continue long after the moment in 1984 when Ned and Felix's relationship stops. Rather than bringing *The Normal Heart* to closure, Felix's death gives Kramer the space to promote an activist agenda once more. Ned recommits himself to an activist career—to the creation of change—a move that reapplies a subversive edge to a play that showed considerable signs of ending its ideological work in the service of a bourgeois status quo.

Although at first glance a seemingly incongruous add-on to the play, Ned's final speech can also be understood in terms of the recommitment to activism that Felix's death allows. Although *The Normal Heart* is rife with anomalous statements and occurrences, Ned's recollection of a gay dance he attended at Yale seems particularly out of place, something even he realizes would have been more appropriate to bring up while Felix was alive. Wondering aloud to his brother Ben why he didn't "fight harder" to save Felix's life, Ned suddenly changes the subject and begins speaking to Felix:

> . . . I forgot to tell him something. Felix, when they invited me to Gay Week at Yale, they had a dance . . . In my old college dining hall, just across the campus from that tiny freshman room where I wanted to kill myself because I thought I was the only gay man in the world—they had a dance. Felix, there were six hundred young men and women there. Smart, exceptional young men and women. Thank you, Felix. (pp. 122-123; second ellipsis in original)

Why Kramer would end his play with such a seemingly insignificant recollection makes little sense until one views it within the context of *The Normal Heart*'s almost frantic attempt to reestablish its commitment to activism in the remaining minutes after Felix dies. Even in those instances in which it has ostensibly depicted the activities of the AIDS organization, *The Normal Heart,* up to this point, has made its primary narrative and ideological commitments to the story of an individual (usually Ned) or a couple (usually Ned and Felix).[27] Ned's reference to the dance at Yale, however, represents a significant (albeit last-ditch) attempt to reverse this pattern through the articulation of a vision of community and collective action. Such a reversal occurs in two ways. First, Ned's discovery of a community of hundreds of gay men and lesbians upon returning to Yale stands in sharp contrast with his previous experience of his homosexuality there as one of isolation. Second, the fact that these men and women are in college is significant as well, for as such, they represent the next generation of political activists—the "exceptional" men and women who will pick up the struggle when Ned's generation has tired or died. By displacing *The Normal Heart*'s previous emphasis on the individual and the couple, then, Ned's speech gestures to the kind of collective work that groups such as ACT UP and GMHC have realized is essential for an effective response to AIDS. Even if, as Crimp and others have argued, Ned's *experience* of activism is considerably more individualistic than collective, Ned's final speech offers a *vision* of the future that is largely communitarian in nature.[28]

ANGELS IN AMERICA

For all its appearances of radicalism, Tony Kushner's *Angels in America* revolves around the kind of realistically rendered love story that is such a central component of *The Normal Heart*. In fact, whereas the title of the play comes from a number of magical scenes in which angels engage in lyrical philosophizing about the state of the world and the nature of human progress, the play's more realistic (and I would argue more compelling) scenes have to do with the collapse and/or formation of three couples: Prior Walter, a caterer with AIDS, and Louis Ironson, his word-processor boyfriend; Joe Pitt, chief clerk for a federal appeals judge (as well as a protégé of Roy Cohn), and Harper, his Valium-addicted wife; and a third couple that forms when Louis and Joe leave their respective partners and enter a relationship with each other.

Significantly, both detractors and supporters of *Angels in America* have identified the story of its couples as the play's dramatic core. Reviewing *Millennium Approaches* for *Time* magazine, for instance, William A. Henry III argued that *"Angels* has indeed electrified reviewers with its radical political perspective and literary style, but is at heart a fairly conventional drama about the intersections of three households in turmoil."[29] Likewise, Michael Feingold made a similar (albeit it more critical) comment in the *Village Voice,* pointing to the extent to which Kushner's attention to his character's intersecting love lives deliberately pandered to mainstream audiences. "If one leaves out the dense texture," Feingold noted, ". . . the play boils down to a simple, faintly sentimental, story: Two guys love each other; one panics when he learns the other has AIDS; after much travail he comes back. This makes a nice *haimisha* evening for Broadway liberals."[30] Such a critical privileging of *Angels in America*'s domestic dramas over its more experimental scenes should not be entirely surprising, of course, given the extent to which the romance narratives in Kushner's play represent the kinds of familiar stories with which any audience member could easily identify.

Angels in America is also centrally concerned with politics, however, and two important processes that I have located in *The Normal Heart* also occur in Kushner's play. First, in order to maintain its mainstream appeal while still promoting political change, *Angels in America* waffles in its decision of whether to embrace its love plot or its politics plot. In fact, the exact nature of this waffling process resembles what we saw in *The Normal Heart:* Although siding at first with its love plot, *Angels in America* does a quick about-face at the end, breaking up its couples so that the play can regain its political voice. Second, as was the case with Ned Weeks, the movement of *Angels in America* between love and politics is paralleled by a similar metamorphosis on the part of a major character—in this case, Louis.

Angels in America's initial embrace of romance, and its concurrent marginalization of political struggle, occurs on two levels. On a "macro" level, the play as a whole devotes most of its attentions to the coming together and breaking apart of its three couples, sacrificing its polemic potential in favor of bourgeois convention. On a "micro" level, this process is paralleled by the events of Joe and Louis's relationship itself. Since Louis's relationship with Prior and Joe's marriage to Harper are on the brink of collapse even as the play begins (Louis leaves Prior when the latter discovers he has AIDS, while Joe leaves Harper upon acknowledging he is gay), the process of courtship and coupling that is central to the love story in literature really belongs to Joe and Louis. Lonely and guilt-wracked after his breakup with Prior, Louis abandons politics for love, jettisoning his noticeably liberal credentials in order to enter into a relationship with a Reaganite Mormon.

Although their first night of sex together represents a bigger personal step for Joe than for Louis, Louis's continued involvement with Joe requires a major shift in his mind-set as well. Up until this point in the play, Louis has served, as David Savran has noted, as the mouthpiece for a liberal pluralist politics—albeit one grounded much more in theory than in practice.[31] At one point in the play, in fact, Louis even assembles a damning indictment of the nastier, more Republican side of bourgeois liberalism, the side that leaves oppressed groups such as gays behind when the going gets rough, and his comments take on particular significance in light of what turns out to be Joe's subscription to just such a politics. "These people [Jeane Kirkpatrick, George Bush] don't begin to know what, ontologically, freedom is or human rights," Louis complains:

> like they see these bourgeois property-based Rights-of-Man-type rights but that's not enfranchisement, not democracy, not what's implicit, what's potential within the idea, not the idea with blood in it. That's just liberalism, the worst kind of liberalism, really, bourgeois tolerance, and what I think is that what AIDS shows us is the limits of tolerance, that it's not enough to be tolerated, because when the shit hits the fan you find out how much tolerance is worth. Nothing. And underneath all the tolerance is intense, passionate hatred.[32]

Once he becomes involved with a conservative Republican, however, Louis begins to abandon his politics. Joe and Louis "spend the month in bed,"[33] arguing politics when they're not having sex. "Change is geologically slow," Joe tells Louis. "You must accept that. And accept as rightfully yours the happiness that comes your way" (p. 35), a charge that the guilt-ridden Louis finds difficult to accept at first.

Louis is never in any real danger of adopting Joe's politics for himself, but he takes a significant step away from his previously outspoken positions when he begins to lessen his criticisms of people such as Joe. "Freedom is where we bleed into one another. . . . You will always have to make choices, and finally all life can offer you in the face of these terrible decisions is that you can make the choices freely" (p. 37), Joe argues in relation to both men having left their partners, and Louis finds his resistance to such an argument wavering because of his feelings for Joe. "You seem to be able to live with what you've done," Louis concedes:

> leaving your wife, you're not all torn up and guilty, you've . . . blossomed, but you're not a terrible person, you're a decent, caring man. And I don't know how that's possible, but looking at you it seems to be. You do seem free. (p. 38; ellipsis in original)

Likewise, when Belize attacks Joe's politics later in the play, Louis comes to Joe's defense, guiltily adopting Joe's tactic of distinguishing between types of conservatism. "Joe is a very moral man, he's not even *that* conservative, or . . . well not that *kind* of a . . . ." (p. 95; ellipsis in original). Belize reveals that Joe is a protégé of Roy Cohn, and Louis recoils at the idea. "You think everything is black and white, good and evil, just because somebody is a Republican they're in bed with Roy Cohn. . . . Joe is . . .well, sort of past ideology, not just another lost ineffectual lefty like me, moaning all the time about history and guilt" (p. 95; second ellipsis in original). Louis is eventually swayed by Belize's argument, but not before he has demonstrated a partial willingness to compromise his politics for the sake of love.

Although Louis manages to surprise even himself as he forfeits his liberal credentials ("I'm losing myself in some ideological leather bar" [p. 36], he quips), such a shift in sentiment can be understood as an ideological necessity given the larger project of the play. As was the case in *The Normal Heart,* Louis's swing from polemicist to lover both parallels and enables a shift by the play as a whole from a

challenging polemic to a more conventional love story. Louis abandons his politics, not only because they prove incompatible with his
Republican lover, but also because (as we have seen before) there is
little room to champion a character's commitment to political and
social change in a play that is, if only temporarily, privileging its love
plot. Accordingly, just as Ned's removal from the board of the AIDS
organization puts a temporary stop to both his political ravings and
The Normal Heart's focus on activist politics, Louis' relationship
with a Republican shuts him up as well.

In fact, given the crucial difference that exists in the ways in
which Ned and Louis drop their politics, the love plot in *Angels in
America* is afforded even more emphasis than that in *The Normal
Heart*. On an ideological level, Ned's abandonment of his activist
career creates a space in which he can become a lover (and in which
the play can become a love story), but on a plot level, the cause of
Ned's switch has nothing to do with his budding romance. Rather,
Ned drops his activist career because he is fired from the board of the
AIDS organization. In *Angels in America,* on the other hand, Louis's
abandonment of his progressive politics has *everything* to do with his
falling in (and out of) love: Louis flirts with Joe's neoconservative
philosophy both because it absolves him of responsibility for abandoning his former lover and because an ideological affinity with Joe
is necessary if the relationship between the two men is to succeed.
Besides assuming narrative priority, then, romantic love is actually
represented at this point in the play as worth abandoning one's
politics for, something which *The Normal Heart* never explicitly
concedes.

Although Joe and Louis's coming together is particularly significant, in that it reflects on a microcosmic level the general movement
of Kushner's play away from political struggle and toward love,
Kushner develops his rather complicated love plot in other ways as
well. As soon as Joe proclaims his love for Louis, Louis realizes he
needs to see Prior again, a realization that devastates Joe. Meanwhile,
Joe, under pressure from Roy Cohn, makes a fainthearted attempt to
return to his wife (in the course of the same evening, Joe has sex with
Harper, tries to see Louis, and then begs Harper to take him back when
he and Louis fight). As such, the central plot question of *Angels in
America* ultimately becomes one of "Who will end up with whom?"

Angels in America, then, like *The Normal Heart,* achieves much of its attractiveness to mainstream audiences through a heavy reliance on the convention of the love story—the inclusion of which requires two things: the displacement of one character's political commitments and the devotion of much of the play's narrative space to its love story (or, in this case, stories). But *Angels in America* resembles *The Normal Heart* in another important way as well. For just as Kramer's play reverses its ideological leanings by its conclusion, so too does *Angels in America* make an about-face in its final scenes, one which again occurs both on a "micro" level (the commitments of an individual character) and a "macro" one (that of the play as a whole). Not only does Louis regain his political footing by rejecting Joe and his reactionary politics, but the play ends up undermining all its love stories in favor of a vision of collectivity and a call for social change.

Kushner ends Joe and Louis's relationship through a reversal of the process that brought them together. Just as Louis shelved his liberal credentials in order to become involved with a Reaganite, so too does his rediscovery of his political rage go hand in hand with his leaving Joe. It is Joe's politics, in fact, that precipitate Louis's change of heart. Having convinced himself earlier in the play that Joe's conservatism could be overlooked, Louis follows up on Belize's information and discovers not only that Joe is in fact a protégé of Roy Cohn, but also that, as a clerk for a mentally incapacitated federal appeals judge, he has penned a series of shockingly reactionary decisions. Most horrifying to Louis is a decision in which a gay member of the army is returned his pension on appeal, but only on a technicality, one which reverses an original decision viewing gays and lesbians as members of a protected class. Here, finally, Joe's Republicanism clashes with the identity politics that underlie Louis's liberalism: although Joe's speeches about individual freedom are at least partially reconcilable with the more libertarian end of Louis's liberalism, his attack on gays demonstrates another side of American conservatism, one which assigns liberal "rights" to some classes of individuals but not to others. When Louis discovers that Joe's past political work has served to disenfranchise a class of people to which he himself belongs, his ability to accommodate Joe's politics collapses.[34]

Besides constituting the moment in the play in which Louis recovers his political sense, Louis's breakup with Joe is also significant in its resemblance to what occurs in an actual activist politics. In the first place, Louis's calling Joe on his court decisions, as well as his refusal to be complicit in them by continuing to be Joe's lover, represents the first instance in *Angels in America* in which Louis's endless political theorizing gets translated into some kind of action. Second, similar to many gay and AIDS activists, Louis literally puts his body on the line: prevented by Louis from leaving the apartment until he has heard what Louis has to say, Joe punches Louis until he collapses—"gay-bashe[d]," as Gordon Rogoff puts it.[35] Third, given Joe's previously undisclosed role as a henchman in the Reagan Revolution, Louis's outraged attack on Joe represents the kind of assault against conservative government players that was the hallmark of AIDS activist politics during the Reagan/Bush years. Thus, although Louis never becomes an activist per se, his breakup with Joe represents the first sign of *Angels in America*'s reorientation toward the kinds of commitments and experiences upon which AIDS activist politics have been grounded in this country.

As a number of critics have pointed out, however, Kushner's resolution of Joe and Louis's relationship is not handled adeptly. Rather, Kushner goes conspicuously out of his way to turn Joe into an emotional monster and an unforgivable reactionary, "assign[ing] him unbelievable lines and motivations" in the words of one reviewer.[36] But although critics have viewed this decision as stemming from Kushner's political disagreements with Republicans, such an explanation is not entirely satisfactory, given that Kushner could have easily changed Joe's politics if he had wanted. In fact, far more plausible than Joe's turning out to be the author of a series of reactionary court decisions would have been the evolution of his politics following his realization that he is gay. Hannah, his mother, starts out equally conservative in *Millennium Approaches,* reacting horribly to her son's homosexuality, but having experienced life in the big city for a while, even she becomes a cosmopolitan New Yorker. No such luck awaits Joe, however, who ends up becoming the scapegoat for all that is wrong in the play (even the heinous Cohn gets treated better).

What I would like to suggest, then, is that Kushner's treatment of Joe is grounded less in his repulsion toward (gay) Republicans than in his need to destroy the central romantic relationship in *Angels in America*. Having served to maintain the interest and empathy of Broadway theatergoers for five hours, Louis and Joe's relationship must nonetheless be terminated if *Angels in America* is to recover its commitment to political struggle. Kushner becomes so intent on eradicating Louis and Joe's relationship—a relationship that has assumed such an important role in the play—that he turns Joe into a monster. Such a move ensures that neither the audience nor Louis will want the relationship to continue, but it also serves to undermine the plausibility of Joe's characterization. As Walter Olson points out, the most glaring example of this is the surprise revelation that Joe has been responsible for writing the offensive court decisions. Put simply, Kushner cheats in this scene: since Joe and Louis have become something of an item, Kushner pulls a rabbit out of a hat, creating a reason for Louis to dump Joe that is understandable in itself, but which makes little sense in terms of the rest of the play. In fact, Louis's sense of betrayal—his cry "You *lied* to me" (p. 111)—is the only moment that makes sense in this scene, for, as Louis realizes, nothing in Joe's previous characterization would have suggested that he was capable of such political mischief (Joe, after all, is the morally uptight lawyer who refuses to help Cohn get the Feds off his back, and who asks the foulmouthed Cohn to "please not take the Lord's name in vain").[37]

Kushner goes even further, however: since Louis is, after all, the character who is able to muster up enough forgiveness to recite Kaddish for Cohn, Kushner ensures that Louis will never be able to forgive Joe for *his* transgressions by having Joe beat him up—even though, as Joe points out, "I never hit anyone before" (p. 112). Unlike Kramer, Kushner does not go so far as to kill off one of his characters in order to end his love story, but both Joe's behavior and the revelations about his past ensure that he will become a persona non grata nonetheless.

Once Louis's breakup with Joe reorients *Angels in America* from romance back to politics on a microlevel, Kushner orchestrates a similar transformation for the play as a whole. Certainly, the possibility of a reconciliation between Joe and Louis seems small (although not impossible) after their violent argument. Nonetheless, with Louis having attempted to "make up" (p. 83) with Prior, and Joe having tried to return to his wife, the collapse of Joe and Louis's relationship in no way signals the end of the love plot in the play. In fact, with so many couple combinations floating around in Kushner's play, audience hopes for "happily ever after" can easily be invested in one of the remaining couples.

The great coup of *Angels in America,* however, is that no one ends up with anyone in the end—at least not in the conjugal sense. Kushner delivers his surprise ending through the use of a split scene showing Louis and Prior in the latter's hospital room and Joe and Harper in their Brooklyn apartment. Harper delivers the bad news first, announcing that she intends to leave. Abandoned by Louis, Joe begs her to stay: "Only you. Only you love me. Out of everyone in the world. I have done things, I'm ashamed. But I have changed" (p. 142), but Harper slaps him across the face in response. Kushner treats Louis's attempt to return to Prior as more of a tease, however, one which relies on audience expectations about what is supposed to happen to divided lovers after they have gained wisdom out in the world. Even if viewers have grown impatient with Joe, who has made many demands on others but has changed little himself, Louis learns and grows from the difficulties he has experienced after leaving Prior. In fact, Louis even manages to fulfill Prior's stated condition for a reconciliation: Prior orders Louis not to return until he can offer "visible scars" (p. 141), rather than mere rhetoric, as a sign of his penitence, a requirement that is strangely fulfilled once Joe assaults Louis.

In fact, although audience expectations about what *should* happen next are initially grounded in literary convention, Kushner fuels these expectations with Prior and Louis's exchange. "I really failed you," Louis admits:

> LOUIS: But . . . this is hard. Failing in love isn't the same as not loving. It doesn't let you off the hook, it doesn't mean . . . you're free to not love.
>
> PRIOR: I love you Louis.
>
> LOUIS: Good. I love you. (p. 143; ellipses in original)

Moreover, in the Broadway production of *Angels in America,* Louis gave physical expression to audience excitement at Prior's revelation that he still loves Louis by collapsing exuberantly into Prior's arms. Having given both Louis and the audience every reason to believe a reconciliation between the two men is possible, however, Prior turns the tables with his next lines:

> **PRIOR:** I really do [love you].
> But you can't come back. Not ever.
> I'm sorry. But you can't. (p. 143)

Such a move is just as a much a rebuke to the audience as it is to Louis, of course. Kushner's refusal to reward Louis and Prior's struggles by allowing them to reunite undermines conventional expectations about what is supposed to happen to a literary couple whose union is rendered impossible by some obstacle at the beginning of the text, but who grow and learn during the course of the play. All that Louis and Prior receive for their pains—and all the audience gets for going on their journey with them—is Prior's refusal to take Louis back.

But although audiences may have expected their reward for sitting through a seven-hour play to be the permanent union of at least one couple (an expectation that is not entirely unreasonable for a play that contains *three* love stories), Kushner offers audiences a different kind of reward instead, one that cannot stand up to the criteria normally applied to bourgeois cultural production. Having managed to eliminate all three of his play's love plots—as well its attendant commitment to bourgeois convention—Kushner turns his full attention to a more communitarian and activist politics, first through a soliloquy that ends the play's final act and then through his epilogue.

Having dismissed the kind of ruthless individualism that formed the basis of Joe's politics, as well as the corollary version of individualism that manifests itself in the bourgeois couple, Kushner offers his audience his first alternative to these ideologies in the play's final scene, as Harper describes the dream she has had while on a flight to San Francisco. Harper is alone in this scene, looking forward to a future separate from her husband. Having severed her ties to New York, and headed to California, she represents on one level the play's final example of a mythic American individualism—a last gasp of the pioneer spirit that pushed people such as Harper's Mormon ancestors west. At the same time, Harper's dream undercuts the individualistic overtones of her venture and contributes further to *Angels in America*'s ideological reorientation. Throughout the play, Harper, who has been going slowly mad from her husband's inattention, has been obsessed by the deterioration of the ozone layer, pointing to it in one scene as an example of the damage being done by Joe's beloved Reagan revolution. Having cast off many of her personal demons in her decision to leave Joe, however, she imagines a collective effort by the earth's dead to repair the damage in the ozone. "Souls were rising, from the earth far below," Harper recounts for the audience:

> souls of the dead, of people who had perished, from famine, from war, from the plague, and they floated up, like skydivers in reverse, limbs all akimbo, wheeling and spinning. And the souls of these departed joined hands, clasped ankles, and formed a web, a great net of souls, and the souls were three-atom oxygen molecules, of the stuff of ozone, and the outer rim absorbed them, and was repaired. (p. 144)

Harper's vision here demonstrates a number of important similarities to Ned's speech at the end of *The Normal Heart*—similarities that point to its important role in reorienting Kushner's play. Most significant, both speeches, although emphasizing the individual on a formal level, are committed to collectivity on the level of content. Both are made by characters whose lives are divorced from the rest of the community (Ned's because of his removal from the board of the AIDS organization, and Harper's because of her decision to leave her husband and her life in New York), and neither are addressed to someone on the stage (Ned "shares" his experience with his dead lover Felix, and Harper's speech is a soliloquy). Nonetheless, the content of each speech belies the experience of the social isolation from which it emanates: both Ned and Harper describe an experience of collectivity and communitarian response, one which, although not actually witnessed by the audience, represents an ideological alternative to the bourgeois individualism upon which the love stories in each play are grounded.

Harper's vision having begun the process, *Angels in America*'s epilogue solidifies the play's move away from the ideological conservatism and stasis of the love story and toward a vision of community, collective struggle, and change. *Angels in America*'s epilogue takes place in February of 1990, four years after the end of the previous act: Prior, Belize, Louis, and Hannah (who befriended Prior earlier in the play) sit together at Bethesda Fountain in Central Park. As usual, Belize and Louis begin arguing about politics, but Prior changes the subject, leading everyone in a group telling of the story of the angel Bethesda, a symbol of the healing and reconciliation that becomes central to the play's final vision.[38] The epilogue then ends with a speech made by Prior to the audience. "This disease will be the end of many of us," Prior proclaims:

> but not nearly all, and the dead will be commemorated and will struggle on with the living, and we are not going away. We won't die secret deaths anymore. The world only spins forward. We will be citizens. The time has come.
>
> Bye now.
>
> You are fabulous creatures, each and every one.
>
> And I bless you: *More Life*.
>
> The Great Work Begins. (p. 148)

Not surprisingly, *Angels in America*'s epilogue has come under attack from a number of critics who have viewed the play's feel-good ending and Prior's blessing of the audience as a sop intended to placate a mainstream Broadway audience.[39] What critics have largely failed to notice, however, is that although Kushner may indeed pander to the audience in his epilogue, he does so while simultaneously undermining bourgeois theatrical convention—and aligning his play with political struggle and change—in two important ways. In the first place, Kushner replaces the couple with the group. As both reviewers and Kushner himself have noted, *Perestroika* is unmistakably a comedy,[40] but it is a comedy that concludes by offering audiences a picture of community rather than the more standard conjugal couple. Even though all three of its couples collapse, *Angels in America* is able to end on a comic note anyway, for its characters are shown to have found sustenance not through the isolative institutions of conjugal marriage or the bourgeois family, but through the benefits of group friendship.[41] Kushner also undermines bourgeois convention by having Prior, Belize, Hannah, and Louis take turns telling the story of the angel Bethesda. For although, as Linda Winer notes in her review of *Millennium Approaches*, the "20 characters" in the first part of the play "never come together in groups larger than duets or the occasional trio,"[42] Kushner's epilogue takes advantage of the ability of drama to effectively represent collectivity, bringing together key characters for what is, in effect, an instance of storytelling as collective action. Although, in conventional terms, *Angels in America* would have been a tragedy of sorts if it had ended with Prior's refusal to allow Louis to return, drama's ability to represent the group allows Kushner to transform his play into a comedy that is grounded in a vision of communal purpose and action.

The second way in which *Angels in America*'s epilogue helps to reverse the ideological leanings of the bulk of the play is through its open ending. Rather than ending his play with Prior's refusal to take Louis back—a move which would have brought it to a tragic version of closure—Kushner reintroduces his major characters in his epilogue, challenging his audience to become agents of social and political change. Prior's companions presage this call through their reference to a number of contemporary political struggles: Louis extols Michael Gorbachev as "the greatest political thinker since Lenin" (p. 145), he makes enthusiastic reference to both the fall of the Berlin Wall and the overthrow of the Ceauşescus in Romania, and he debates the limits of Palestian autonomy with Belize. Prior's own words at the end of the epilogue are what crystallize this sentiment, however. Having offered his elegy for those who have died of AIDS and insisted on the timeliness of full citizenship for gays, Prior repeats the words the angel spoke over his bed at the end of *Millennium Approaches*: "The Great Work Begins." But while the appearance of this line at the end of *Millennium Approaches* suggested that it was Prior who was to be the agent of important change, Kushner's reinsertion of these words at the end of *Perestroika* indicates that the agent of this "great work" must be the audience itself. As such, I would argue that the epilogue of *Angels in America* be read as a call for activism: having offered audiences both a denunciation of Reaganism and a vision of community and collective action, Kushner instructs them that the process of social change he envisions is not an imaginative process, but rather one that can only "begin" once the play itself has ended.

CONCLUSION

Given the distinctions that critics are beginning to draw between "first" and "second generation" AIDS plays, I find it significant that *Angels in America* and *The Normal Heart* possess the structural and ideological similarities that I have outlined in this chapter. What has remained the same between 1985 and 1993 is the dilemma that politically committed writers such as Kramer and Kushner have faced in representing the epidemic. In light of the hold that the love story in literature has on the popular imagination, both Kramer's and Kushner's decision to organize their respective plays around romantic love must be viewed as a logical and highly strategic move. Likewise, given their personal histories as AIDS activists, the decision of both of these playwrights to include—and ultimately champion—political struggle in their plays is entirely understandable as well. But despite the logic of including both plot lines in these plays, love and political struggle prove ultimately incompatible.

Angels in America and *The Normal Heart* are not the only imaginative texts that have difficulty balancing narratives of love and politics. In fact, one need only think of the novels discussed in Chapter 2 for additional examples. In Monette's *Afterlife,* for instance, the closure attendant with the love story involving Mark and Steven ("the sleepers had all they needed") creates a situation in which political struggle (represented by Dell) must be displaced from the text. Conversely, in the case of *People in Trouble,* Schulman is forced to end Kate's relationship with both Peter and Molly so that her novel can conclude with a call for continued political action.[43]

The conflict that I have focused on most in this chapter—that between erotic love and political struggle—is heavily dependent on Kramer's and Kushner's use of traditional literary forms, a choice adopted by Monette and Schulman as well. Whether falling into the categories of realism (Kramer), social realism (Schulman), magic realism (Kushner), or quasi-utopian fiction (Monette), all of the novels and plays discussed in this book possess similar qualities: They are organized around narrative lines that are roughly chronological, run through the entire text, and move toward (even if sometimes rejecting) closure; they contain characters who act in a logical fashion and are able to produce an empathetic reaction among readers and viewers; and they avoid calling attention to themselves stylistically, thereby highlighting content. Although love and politics might be able to cohabitate in more experimental kinds of fiction and drama, this chapter has focused on the problems that occur in including both of these plot lines in more traditional texts—i.e., in the kinds of writing that have an extensive appeal to mainstream audiences.[44]

But although the structural limitations of traditional fiction and drama contribute to this conflict, these limitations can be traced back one step further to a long-standing ideological conflict between the private and the public in the Western political imagination. What makes the way that these conflicts play themselves out in the writings of Monette, Kushner, Kramer, and Schulman so interesting, however, is the extent to which AIDS wreaked havoc upon this long-standing ideological division, turning profoundly private acts into matters of public concern—among public health officials, AIDS educators, and gay men advocating for state mobilizations against the epidemic.[45]

What the writers I have examined in this book come up against, in other words, is a paradoxical situation in which the traditional literary forms they use to create an imaginative response to AIDS have no way of keeping up with the collapse between the public and the private engendered by the very epidemic they chronicle (a collapse of which all of them seem more or less aware). Just as gay men have been ambivalent about giving up their positioning within the dominant classes, they have also proven ambivalent about abandoning this crucial liberal distinction between public and private. Accordingly, a writer such as Paul Monette can end up advocating a *private* resolution to the problem of AIDS, even though the isolation of private life from the concerns of the world has been rendered impossible by the epidemic. Likewise, a writer such as Larry Kramer might side with a public response to AIDS at the end of his play, but only after holding on to the possibility of a distinctly private one for as long as possible. Since many gay men have benefited (both economically and socially) from the distinction between the private and the public, choosing to keep their gay identities a private matter, the writings of these men evidence a profound ambivalence about the need to give up this distinction.[46]

Given the extent to which AIDS is a disease that closely binds eros and politics—the private and the public—the inability of traditional drama and fiction to integrate both proves all the more unfortunate. As we shall see in the next chapter, this binding process was one of which many AIDS activists were themselves acutely aware. In contrast to the imaginative literature of the epidemic, however, these activists were often quite successful at integrating eros and politics in their work, thereby collapsing the public/private distinction that circumscribes the political work performed by these texts.

Chapter 4

ACT UP as Gay Politics

We used to do benefits every now and again . . . and we'd
go to a bar, and take it over for the night, and dance
around, and sell T-shirts and stuff. And my cheeks would
hurt the next day because I'd spent the whole night laugh-
ing and smiling, and I just really felt like I had found
where I belonged.

—Bill Jesdale, ACT UP/RI

ACT UP was a big meat market.

—Sarah Schulman, ACT UP/New York

Ever since its creation in 1987, ACT UP has been the subject of
a number of public controversies. Most of these stemmed from
ACT UP's infamous tactics: the group is probably most famous for
its 1989 "Stop the Church" demonstration, which generated news
coverage (and denunciation) worldwide after a group of activists
disrupted mass inside St. Patrick's Cathedral while thousands of
others protested outside. Tactics aside, however, ACT UP was also
the target of another line of criticism, one stemming from the tricky
relationship between gay politics and AIDS politics in the United
States. Beginning in the late 1980s, ACT UP found itself attacked
from two opposing sides—while some commentators viewed it as
being too gay, others complained that it was not gay enough.

On the one hand, a number of ACT UP's detractors argued that
the group's focus on AIDS distracted its members from the real

needs of the gay community. Darrell Yates Rist generated extensive controversy with a 1989 *Nation* article castigating the lesbian and gay community for its "obsession" with AIDS at the expense of other community projects, such as antiviolence work or the provision of services for gay teens. These projects, Rist argued, would involve building up the gay community rather than focusing on its demise. Rist reserved particularly harsh language for ACT UP, which he accused of propagating "this panicky faith that all of us are doomed," and he was equally critical of what he viewed as the tendency of "these AIDS crusaders" (ACT UP and GMHC partisans alike) to "never go public over the right of homosexuals to something more than not dying."[1] Furthermore, in a response to letters in a later issue of *The Nation* critical of his article, Rist accused "the AIDS-devout" of managing to "scare the libido out of a citizenry more thoroughly than legal proscriptions have ever managed to, successfully executing the office of collaborators."[2]

Robin Hardy made a related argument in a *Village Voice* article in 1991, suggesting that ACT UP's politics were threatening the gay community by contributing to a general " 'de-gaying' of AIDS activism." By focusing so much attention on the AIDS-related needs of women and minorities (especially those needs resulting from the effects of "racism and sexism"), ACT UP had managed to marginalize the needs of HIV-positive gay men, Hardy claimed. "As ACT UP embraces the politics of inclusion," he warned, "it cuts itself off from the community which has provided the core of its tactics, theory, membership, and funding."[3]

Clearly, Hardy's critique of ACT UP here is very different from Rist's, but what united the two pieces was a shared perception that ACT UP was increasingly failing to act in the best interests of the gay (and particularly the gay male) community.

Paradoxically, a second line of criticism took ACT UP to task for *too* much focus on the needs of the gay community—a position viewed as inappropriate for an organization claiming to be a "diverse" coalition focused on the needs of all populations with HIV. For instance, in a *Village Voice* article on ACT UP's disruption of Health and Human Services Secretary Louis Sullivan's speech at the 1990 International Conference on AIDS in San Francisco, Frank Browning found himself torn over the demonstration's effects.

While praising the protest for "demonstrating gay power in the time of AIDS to gay people," Browning questioned the symbolic significance (as well as the underlying reality) of a group of mostly white AIDS activists choosing the speech of an African-American male as the only speech to interrupt during the entire conference (a significance only partially offset, in Browning's opinion, by the positioning of black and Latino members of ACT UP at the front of the demonstration). Interrupting Sullivan's speech, Browning argued, "was certainly not about building common cause with all of the diverse populations struggling against the epidemic." ACT UP might give lip service to the AIDS-related needs of women, poor people, and people of color, Browning insisted, but it should not and could not speak on behalf of those groups.[4]

An analysis of ACT UP's social side can provide us with one way of reconciling the conflicting lines of criticism I have just outlined. What analyses such as Rist's, Hardy's, and Browning's ignored—what most commentary on ACT UP ignores, in fact—is the extremely important role that socializing among members played for ACT UP. Although most observers of the group saw only rowdy demonstrations, an equally important part of the ACT UP experience was the dating, sex, friendship, and community formation that occurred between and among members. This social activity, I would argue, represented one way in which ACT UP made an important intervention into gay (as opposed to AIDS) politics in this country—whether in a large chapter such as ACT UP/New York or a smaller chapter such as ACT UP/RI. Although ACT UP's activism was necessarily focused on AIDS, its social side was all about being gay.[5]

DRESS LIKE YOU WOULD FOR A DATE

Toward the end of my fieldwork with ACT UP/New York, I violated my own rule concerning the level of actual involvement I would have in the organization. Although I had been told throughout the summer that ACT UP was considerably less factionalized than it had been just a few years earlier, competing philosophical camps were still very much in evidence, and I had decided that the best way to get to talk to the most people would be to avoid taking a public position on any divisive issue. As such, I generally bit my lip during the heated debates that peppered Monday night meetings. By August, however, I had become heavily involved in a committee working on legalizing needle possession, and when no one else expressed interest in presenting to "the floor" our committee's idea for a demonstration, I volunteered. ACT UP/RI had usually been willing to put its name behind any AIDS-related activity that someone was willing to take the time to organize, but demonstrations in ACT UP/New York were a much harder sell, and a more experienced member of our committee suggested that I consult with her before I made my pitch to the floor. I called her up and was given some suggestions on the handout I had put together to explain the demonstration, but then I was offered a more important piece of advice: "Dress like you would for a date," I was told.

I relay this anecdote as a means of beginning my analysis, for I find it richly suggestive of the extent to which sex and sexuality, dating and friendship, socializing, and community formation shaped both ACT UP's identity as an organization and the involvement of individual members. I first encountered this intersection of the personal and the political in ACT UP shortly after joining ACT UP/RI. Although I myself had originally come to ACT UP in part as a means of meeting other gay people, in time I began to find the social component of the group a little overbearing—a "distraction" from the political work I had assumed would be the central focus of an AIDS activist organization. "Wasn't the purpose (or at least the primary purpose) of ACT UP supposed to be AIDS activism?" I began asking myself.

During my three months with ACT UP/New York in 1993, I discovered a similar level of social activity, although one with a much larger sexual component than what had existed in ACT UP/RI. Facilitators would frequently have to ask those in attendance on Monday nights to refrain from chatting during meetings, and in good weather, people would wander out to the garden at the Lesbian and Gay Community Center to smoke and talk with friends during parts of the meeting they found uninteresting. Arduous tasks such as poster making were turned into all-day, drop-in "parties," and dinner excursions often followed Monday night meetings or the meetings of committees (however, the size of ACT UP/New York—as well as serious internal divisions—precluded the kind of whole-group excursions I was familiar with in ACT UP/RI). Still, I was told that the level of social activity I observed in ACT UP/New York was but a mere shadow of what had existed just a few years earlier, when hundreds of new members had flocked to ACT UP, attracted by its increasingly "in" reputation, forcing it to move Monday night meetings to the larger auditorium in Cooper Union. "Cooper Union's an enormous auditorium," B.C. Craig recalled:

> It's one of the largest auditoriums in New York, and it was packed with people. And most of them weren't sitting in their seats: most of them were walking around in the background, hanging out. And a lot of that was little groups of people meeting and stuff like that. But a lot of it was just an enormous amount of socializing going on. Networking. And it seemed to me like hardly anyone was paying any attention to the meeting. I had never been in a group like that before, where people didn't seem to be focused on what was going on.

As might be expected, important differences existed in the patterns and meanings of social activity in ACT UP/New York and ACT UP/RI. For instance, although dating among members occurred in both chapters, New York activists I talked to were much more likely than their Rhode Island counterparts to cite the potential for sexual and romantic interactions among members as an important draw for the organization. "[In] '89, '90, people were dating each other like crazy," Stephen Gendin recalled. "I mean, there was an ACT UP slumber party once at the [Lesbian and Gay] Community Center. . . . I don't know if there was any particular point to it other than a social thing, but there were like a hundred people, and it turned into an all-night orgy." Writer and activist Sarah Schulman had a similar recollection: "ACT UP was a big meat market, and that was one of its biggest recruitment things. Every sexy boy from a certain generation came through ACT UP at some point or another."

Some New York activists suggested, in fact, that given the amount of time many people put into the organization and the shared perspective that drew members together, it was inevitable that romantic interests would arise between members. "These are people I can relate to on many levels, other than just merely sexually," Norberto Stuart (NYC) explained. "So, if I were looking for more than a fuck—than a trick—I would most likely end up developing feelings for someone within ACT UP." Stuart also indicated that his HIV-positive status played an important role in this realization. "I've had sexual partners whom I have liked a lot as people," he noted:

> but I don't feel that it can transcend the fuck buddy part, simply because they're not politically informed, or concerned. And so here's a person who doesn't know my status, and really isn't interested or invested in the AIDS arena, so how can I share all of me as a person with them, when it would most likely either scare them or it would just be something that they wouldn't want to become invested in? Whereas in ACT UP, the men are, if not positive themselves, at least perhaps not totally nauseated by the prospect of being intimate with me, and I come to know them as people and what their agendas are.

Sex was such an important entity in ACT UP/New York, in fact, that even political activity was described in sexual terms. A popular action that would grab a lot of media attention was considered "sexy," while strong-arm tactics would sometimes be necessary to get people to participate in a demonstration that did not fit the bill. An unappealing demonstration could be made sexier, however, if it was presented in a sufficiently sexy manner—thus the advice to "dress like you would for a date."

It is important to note that not everyone in ACT UP/New York found dating opportunities to be so plentiful. Especially if they had joined ACT UP later in its history, women tended to feel that the potential for meeting partners was much smaller for them than it was for the men, given the smaller number of women in the organization. When asked about her own experience with dating in ACT UP, for example, Mary Cotter contrasted her current situation with what she had encountered upon first joining in 1992. "Only if somebody new walks in, then it's a serious cruising ground. We're all climbing over each other to get to her!" Cotter noted. "But no, there are no women there. When I first came, it was [a cruising ground], because I didn't know anyone, but now I know all twenty women." Activists also suggested that, although men had historically come to ACT UP to look for dates, women tended not to. Schulman pointed out, for instance, that since ACT UP/New York was such a male-dominated organization, women who would even consider joining the group tended to do so because they were already seriously committed to progressive organizing, not because they felt it might provide them with a comfortable environment in which to meet new people. Not all women in ACT UP/New York shared these opinions, however. Trina Johnson, for one, indicated that she found ACT UP/New York's lesbian caucus to be one of the most social units within the organization, and she countered the suggestion that dating opportunities were as rare for women as some had suggested. "There's a lot of cruising that goes on in the room," Johnson noted, "and we pretend that it's happening mostly among the men, but it's actually happening among the women, and across the men and the women."

At the same time that at least some women in ACT UP/New York found dating opportunities less plentiful for them than for the men, however, many of them pointed to the uniqueness for them of belonging to an organization in which gay men and lesbians worked and socialized together. "I lived very much in a lesbian activist ghetto," Craig recalled of her life before joining ACT UP/New York. "I did not know or work with gay men, and I think that ACT UP has been important in changing the gay and lesbian movement forever by bringing gay men and lesbians together in a way that they had never been together before."[6] Johnson described this merger in even stronger terms:

> There's . . . sort of like a sister- and brotherhood between gay men and lesbians. . . . There's sort of that feeling, sort of that camaraderie, like we're not gay *and* lesbian: we are *together.* . . . I think for gay men who want to be around lesbians and lesbians who want to be around gay men, ACT UP is a really nice place to do it, and there are some circles of gay men and lesbians who socialize with each other a lot in ACT UP, who are really tight.

Significantly, such sentiments tended to be expressed mostly by women in the group: if dating opportunities were a social benefit of belonging to ACT UP that represented more of a draw for men than for women, then discovering a space in which lesbians and gay men could work together seemed to have more significance to women members.

ACT UP/RI members often dated among themselves as well; in fact, almost all of the men I interviewed in that group had had a long-term relationship with at least one other member. Nonetheless, activists tended to view ACT UP/RI as a relatively poor environment in which to find lovers, if only because of the group's small size. "I think people who do come . . . for that tend not to stay very long because it doesn't work very well," Bill Jesdale noted, a sentiment that was echoed by other activists. "There were so few members here that after a while you knew everybody," Alan Petrofsky indicated. "We don't get the new boy in town coming to the meeting every now and then."

Much more important to ACT UP/RI members than dating, however, was the degree to which the group's small numbers could create a sense of "family" or "community" for its members.[7] "Every gay person . . . unless they've had a really cool family—which is rare, I think—gets to a point where they realize they need to re-create a sense of community, or family, or however you want to define that," Smith explained, "and I think ACT UP/RI provides that for a certain type of person." Having been a member of *both* ACT UP/New York and ACT UP/RI until 1990, in fact, James McGrath recalled that a sense of organization-wide cohesion was much more possible—and necessary—in a small group such as ACT UP/RI than in the larger New York chapter. "Those ten active people, they were all my friends—everybody in the group I felt a real closeness with," he indicated of ACT UP/RI. "In New York," he added, "it's very confrontational within the group. . . . But if you did that in ACT UP/RI, if you put someone down and took such a personal approach to a negative issue in a meeting, you would probably just break up the whole group as far as I was concerned."

Given the integral nature of ACT UP's social scene to the functioning of the organization as a whole, those who were unable to find a social niche for themselves eventually tended to leave the organization. "It's a strong feeling that people have had," ACT UP/New York's Craig noted:

> that if you are looking for a lover, and there isn't whatever grouping you're looking for available in ACT UP, that people won't stay as long. Or at least, if there isn't a social group for

you, then people don't stay. Which is why we've lost most of the straight people, a lot of older people. ACT UP has become a sort of twenties, early thirties group—a pretty homogeneous bunch.

Jesdale offered a similar explanation for ACT UP/RI's being mostly white gay men. "If you don't fit into the social scene of ACT UP," he noted:

> then it's very hard to get involved in the other aspect of it too, because every subcommittee meeting is at someone's house, and is sort of this social event. Which is a great way to do business, but which also leaves people who aren't feeling like they're part of that social scene left out.

Ann Kraft (RI) echoed Jesdale's assessment, indicating that she had failed to find a sufficient level of emotional support in the dinner excursions that followed ACT UP/RI's weekly meetings. Although "people were friends and socialized, which is usually a mechanism for dealing with emotions," Kraft recalled, she felt distanced from such a therapeutic outlet as a heterosexual woman:

> I kind of felt like [laughs] I was not one of the guys. . . . The fact that I'm a woman, and the fact that I'm straight, or mostly straight, puts this kind of difference there. . . . Because guys were talking about who they wanted to sleep with, or if they had a boyfriend, or not—life stuff, whatever, gossip. I was much further outside of that.

Dating and friendships within ACT UP occurred outside of public view, and it is easy to view them as peripheral to ACT UP's activist politics. Nonetheless, the very existence of such activity goes a long way in defending ACT UP from the kinds of criticisms I outlined earlier. When ACT UP members found friends, lovers, or a sense of family within that organization, they participated in a kind of political work that bridged the gap between gay and AIDS politics. Socializing served an important political function within ACT UP, for it assisted members in creating a community experience that was distinctly different from what other gay organizations had to offer.

For instance, although New York City provided ACT UP/New York members with numerous outlets for finding some version of a community experience, activists cited important differences between the kinds of community available within ACT UP and what they had found in other venues. For one thing, the large amount of dating that occurred among members of ACT UP/New York helped to create a uniquely politicized community experience, one that might be understood as a putting into practice of many of ACT UP's politics concerning AIDS and sex. ACT UP was always committed to a response to AIDS based on safer sex practices rather than abstinence, but it combined this pro-sex stance with a continual insistence that the community put AIDS at the front of its agenda. "Especially in a time when gay bars and baths had such a bad reputation because of the scare of AIDS," Craig explained, "ACT UP was a place that you could go and be sexy and sociable and still feel like you were dealing with the crisis instead of denying it. And so, ACT UP has always had a real history of a lot of sexual dynamics going on."

ACT UP created a venue in which members could be openly sexual with one another, in which no one expected that an HIV diagnosis would stop a person from taking lovers, in which asking a partner for safe sex was a norm—and in which the presence of AIDS was never forgotten. In a combination that in other contexts might actually seem morbid, meetings created a space in which the undisguised opportunity to meet potential lovers coexisted with activism concerning a deadly disease. In an ACT UP context, such a combination made complete sense, for ACT UP was as committed to calling attention to the reasons why gay men were dying as it was to the continued promotion of free sexual expression within the gay community. To observers such as Rist, however, who saw only ACT UP's activist side (its "obsession" with AIDS), ACT UP was viewed as "scar[ing] the libido out of a citizenry more thoroughly than legal proscriptions have ever managed to." But such an analysis failed to take into consideration half the picture of what ACT UP did, for ACT UP functioned as a microcommunity in which an "obsession" with AIDS could coexist with a continuous celebration—and actualization—of a type of active sexual expression threatened by the epidemic. During a decade in which politicians and public health officials attempted to curtail other channels for gay sexuality (and often succeeded), or in which segments of the gay community viewed AIDS as too much of a "downer" to address, ACT UP's combination of the two became a political project in itself.

A second way in which ACT UP/New York created community for members was by serving as a community of shared opinion—a gay community of sorts, certainly, but one whose views and priorities positioned it outside of mainstream gay and lesbian life. As Gendin pointed out, for instance, although most ACT UP/New York members had extensive contact with gays outside of the organization, one reason why they had joined ACT UP was to be with lesbians and gay men who shared a point of view that was hard to find in the rest of the community. "You were involved with ACT UP/New York not because you didn't have gay friends," Gendin explained, "but because your other gay friends might be bankers who were just perfectly happy to go and make $100,000 a year . . . and within ACT UP/New York you found a group of people who really had a similar sense of urgency and time frame and political view point." John Weir recalled things similarly. "I remember a time—I guess in '91—when I was going [to ACT UP] where I always felt like it was the one place I could be where people had the same understanding of the world that I had." ACT UP/New York members, in fact, were often quick to disparage the political priorities of the rest of the gay community. During the summer I spent with the group, a number of members voiced disdain for several projects: the wearing of red ribbons to express support for people with AIDS, the energy and dollars the community (and especially some of its most prominent members) had plunged into the fight over gays in the military, and the mainstreaming politics exhibited at the 1993 March on Washington.

Given the important differences that existed between gay life in Rhode Island and that in major urban areas, both the kinds of community created within ACT UP/RI and the political work done by such community formation varied considerably from what existed in ACT UP/New York. Although members of both chapters pointed to the importance of friendships and community within their organizations, Rhode Island activists in particular viewed their chapter as providing members with needed support in a homophobic and largely closeted state.[8] In fact, members who had moved to Rhode Island from other cities suggested that ACT UP/RI more than other

ACT UP chapters served this particular function. Petrofsky indicated, for instance, that although being surrounded by gay people at work and in the evenings lessened his need for the social side of ACT UP while he lived in New York, the situation became very different when he moved to Rhode Island. "In Rhode Island," he explained, "I come here [ACT UP] because here I'm surrounded by straight people all day, and basically a heterosexual world, and so I come here and it's a gay world. I didn't need that in New York, because my life was a gay world." Likewise, upon coming to Rhode Island as a student after doing work with ACT UP/DC, M. Moore Robinson sensed that ACT UP/RI was playing the role of a support group as much as an activist organization. "The general idea I got," Robinson explained:

> was that in Rhode Island, dealing with homophobia and AIDS-phobia was at so much more a basic level than the other communities I've been in . . . there seemed to be the issue of finding people who you could be out and gay with, and *that* was a remarkable occurrence in Rhode Island.

ACT UP/RI, Robinson felt, provided members with "a way of being able to identify as gay in a safe place."

Other venues for finding gay people certainly existed in Rhode Island—ranging from bars, to social groups, to a number of high-visibility political organizations—and ACT UP members were no strangers to these community spaces. Nonetheless, ACT UP/RI members (like their New York counterparts) understood their organization as an alternative space, one that could provide a different type of community experience than that available elsewhere. For one thing, members often distinguished themselves from other gay Rhode Islanders in terms of their self-understanding of what it meant to be gay—an understanding organized around the politics of being out of the closet. In a state in which many gay people tended to remain extremely closeted, Robinson noted, "drawing attention to us was disrupting the plans of people who were in the closet and liked to stay that way." In fact, ACT UP/RI's high-visibility profile provides a partial explanation for why, in a state that draws relatively few lesbian and gay newcomers, most ACT UP members were not Rhode Island natives: lacking in-state ties, members had more leeway to be open about their sexuality. As ACT UP/RI member Peter Hocking explained, "They [activists from out of state] don't have to worry about parents, or friends of the family, or anyone seeing this on television—it's not going to be broadcast in Wyoming."

Members also pointed to their political stands as something that distinguished them from other gays in the state. "These were students who were very active as gay students at RISD [Rhode Island School of Design] or Brown, but who were angry enough that they weren't finding on a *political* level gay people that they connected with," recalled Gendin, who helped to found ACT UP/RI in 1988 after a period of work with ACT UP/New York. "So yes, in some senses, it was a support group of gay people with a similar mentality." As in ACT UP/New York, then, social activity within ACT UP/RI played a pronounced political role. By providing members with a sense of community in a homophobic environment, and by creating a supportive environment for a group of people whose identity and politics found little affirmation in the rest of the state, ACT UP/RI was able to expand its political impact well beyond its activism.

Community formation within ACT UP is a geographically specific process, and the differences between the kinds of social opportunities cultivated within ACT UP/RI and ACT UP/New York can be understood in terms of the political and social climate within which each group operated. For instance, the localized needs of the New York gay community provide a partial explanation for why dating among members was so much more common in—and seen as much more important to—ACT UP/New York than ACT UP/RI. ACT UP/RI operated in an AIDS climate in which a much smaller percentage of gay men were HIV infected than in New York, and in which needle sharing played a disproportionate role in HIV transmission. Historically, relatively few ACT UP/RI members were themselves HIV positive (or at least openly so), and the generalized effects of homophobia (such as a basic fear of coming out) represented a greater threat to gay existence in the state than did sexually transmitted diseases. In New York, however, the situation was very different. Historically, up to 50 percent of the gay men in the city have been estimated to be infected with HIV, and sex between men has always been a primary means of HIV transmission there. Given a climate, then, in which the threat of AIDS to gay male sex has represented such a central challenge to the gay community, ACT UP/ New York's endorsement of a pro-sex politics, combined with its creation of a space in which members (and especially men) could readily meet lovers, directly responded to the needs of the gay community in that city. As such, New York activists cited the importance of sex and dating within ACT UP far more often than did their Rhode Island counterparts.

However, given that ACT UP/RI operated in a state where homophobia and gay isolation were much more common than in New York City, Rhode Island activists cited mutual support, a sense of community, and—most important—group cohesion as the most valuable benefits of belonging to ACT UP, and they adjusted their political work accordingly. Conflicts and squabbles certainly occurred in the organization, but since one of the purposes of ACT UP/RI was to create a united front against *outside* opposition (from both hostile straights and more conservative gays), it eschewed much of the infighting that New York activists often accepted as an inevitable part of grassroots politics, especially during its early years. At the same time, Rhode Island activists expressed little regret over the relative lack of dating opportunities available in that chapter, faced as they were with the more pressing need of providing support for one another.

CONCLUSION

By focusing in this chapter on ACT UP's social component—a part of ACT UP that most analyses ignore, but which was of central importance to the organization—I have tried to suggest a means of responding to critiques of ACT UP's relationship to gay politics. Dating and friendships within ACT UP must be understood not only as an interesting sidebar to the activism, but also as important political projects in themselves, ones in which processes of community formation both addressed the needs of gay and lesbian members and made political interventions into the larger gay community and society at large. The centrality of social activity within ACT UP represents a challenge to Rist and others like him who felt that ACT UP abandoned projects that built up the gay community in favor of an "obsession" with the community's demise. Likewise, Hardy's 1991 assertion that ACT UP had turned away from the needs of gay men strikes me as a questionable way of describing the organization at a time when social activity within ACT UP was at its greatest peak, and when the social needs of gay men were addressed by ACT UP far more than those of any other group. Hardy was focused on AIDS-related needs, of course, but as I have demonstrated in this chapter, the creation of sexual opportunities and communities of support—although by no means a replacement for treatments or a cure—constituted political projects in themselves at a time when gay male sexuality and identity were under attack.

My analysis here also provides a partial explanation for why ACT UP remained a gay organization, even as the demographics of the epidemic shifted to include an increasing number of heterosexuals. Critiques such as Browning's suggest that as long as ACT UP's membership was primarily gay, it was unable to address the needs of communities in which AIDS affects many (although not necessarily mostly) heterosexuals—if not because ACT UP is insensitive to the needs of these communities, then because these communities will want to organize on their own behalf. But although the inclusion of more heterosexuals (white and nonwhite alike) might have assisted ACT UP in shaping the politics of AIDS during a time of changing epidemic demographics, attempts to include straights proved historically unsuccessful, in part because of ACT UP's additional commitment to responding to the social needs of gay men and lesbians. ACT UP remained a gay organization not because members were unaware of the exigencies of a changing epidemic, but because it served an important function within gay as well as AIDS politics, a function that members came to count on from the organization. Although the presence of more heterosexuals would have been unlikely to interfere with dating, friendships, and community formation among gay and lesbian activists, such a presence was unlikely so long as socializing among gays remained a central and institutionalized component of the organization.

Not to mention one that was, in the final analysis, closely tied to ACT UP's activist agenda. "I would say that actually the passion fuels us, that passion and desire keep us going," Trina Johnson reminded me when I asked her if all the socializing within ACT UP/ New York ever distracted from the activism:

We want to keep having sex, we want to keep being queer, we want to keep shooting up, or having choices available to us, you know? And seeing people we can fuck right in front of us almost makes you want to say, "This is really important, I want to live this way, I've got to be able to continue living, and so I've got to work on these issues." And it's important, these are people I care about dying, or potentially getting infected. I forget a lot of times that some of the people I love and am really close with as an activist on the floor are HIV positive, and when I remember that it's just all of a sudden like, "POW!! I can never stop working on this issue." . . . That has to keep you going, too.

Appendix

Research Methodology

Oral historians, as Michael Frisch has noted, must constantly grapple with the crucial question, "What happens to experience on the way to becoming memory?"[1] In Chapters 1 and 4 of this book, I have used the words of ACT UP members as oral evidence that, however subjective, could provide a layer of factual information upon which to build my analysis, and I have treated my interviews as no better or worse forms of evidence than written documents.[2] At the same time, oral history interviews *are* a unique kind of evidence in a variety of respects, and it is worth considering what the kinds of interviews I conducted, as well as their dependence on the personal experiences of activists, can and cannot tell us about ACT UP.

Oral historians have generally agreed that one of the most important aspects of their craft is that it has allowed them to give "voice to the voiceless"—to record the experiences of people who have not left written records, or whose ideas and contributions have traditionally been ignored.[3] ACT UP, however, was hardly voiceless. In fact, the group was largely organized around the idea of publicity: it had a sophisticated media committee that constantly churned out evidence of its existence; its committees produced dozens of documents a week; and it spent much of its time organizing activities that would garner newspaper and television coverage. Nor has ACT UP failed to leave behind a written record: ACT UP/New York had a huge archives that is now in the possession of the New York Public Library, and ACT UP/RI's own archives are now part of the Special Collections Department of the Brown University Library (currently housed in the John Hay Library).[4]

Nonetheless, oral history interviewing remained a crucial part of my research on ACT UP, not because there were no other documents available, but because I was centrally concerned with a series of problems about which I was convinced the written record would have little to say. Media accounts of ACT UP demonstrations had little insight into the kinds of behind-the-scenes activism that I knew to be an essential part of ACT UP's work; moreover, ACT UP's endless stream of official publications tended to downplay internal conflicts and crises facing the organization. As such, I realized, oral histories would be essential to my project.[5]

Memory is obviously an extremely subjective kind of historical document, but my project in this study was one that I feel was not harmed by, and may in fact have benefited from, the accumulation of such subjective evidence. In the first place, since I was not attempting to write a history of ACT UP, I was generally unconcerned with accumulating hard historical facts, and there are only a few places in this study where I have used the words of an activist to comment on a specific event. Second, and related, subjective evidence was exactly what I was looking for in many cases, since I was often more concerned with ascertaining the *meaning* that ACT UP possessed for activists than with getting down the nitty-gritty details of what happened. Finally, because I had access to dozens of interviews and a number of other kinds of sources, I was able to see places where interpretations and experiences disagreed or clashed, and I have called attention to a number of these disagreements in my analysis.

Dealing with political activists, many of whom had worked and socialized with one another for a number of years, also influenced my interviews in a number of significant ways. As Elizabeth Lapovsky Kennedy and Jane Sherron De Hart have separately noted, oral history interviews have a tendency to veer away from the spontaneous recounting of personal experience and toward the telling of what Kennedy calls "fine-tuned" stories or what De Hart refers to as the "recurring patterns" of "narrative constructions," especially when the experience being recounted is one that occurred in a group context.[6] This insight is extremely applicable to the interviews I draw upon in this study. Women activists especially tended to articulate highly developed analyses of the workings of ACT UP, so much so that it quickly became obvious to me that they had theorized these issues for themselves and talked about them with one another, long before my interviewing began. My interview with Sarah Schulman made this tendency toward narrativizing especially clear: as I began to work on my chapter on Schulman, I found phrases and concepts from my interview with her repeated almost verbatim in her published writings, other published interviews, and even the writings of other ACT UP members. This tendency had two noticeable consequences. First, because of the level of theory and analysis they contained, many of my interviews were able to serve as secondary sources of a sort, as much as "raw" data. Second, even though the focus of my analysis is on white gay men, I have a tendency to quote women activists more than I do the men.[7]

In a similar manner, I was struck by the fact that many activists seemed to return to a party line at times in recounting their experiences. For instance, although most of the ACT UP/New York members I spoke to indicated their support of a joint "inside/outside" approach to politics ("inside" referring to meetings with officials, "outside" to street demonstrations), other written and oral sources suggested that some of these narrators had favored one approach over another.[8] Clearly, some level of consensus had been developed within ACT UP/New York as to what an appropriate grassroots movement would be, and this consensus was reflected in my interviews at times. These tendencies are not altogether surprising, however, since ACT UP was by nature a group in which ideas and tactics were developed collectively and meanings were always shared meanings.

Nor are these tendencies necessarily discouraging. On the one hand, the collective, narrativized nature of much of what I was told means that I probably had less access to the individual experiences of narrators than I had originally imagined. At the same time, since my goal in this study was to develop an analysis of ACT UP as a whole, rather than the experiences of particular individuals, this tendency may simultaneously have cut down on the individual subjectivity of the responses I received. Given the particular nature of my project, in fact, the ability of my interviews to elicit personal experience, received wisdom, and dominant narratives all at once proved extremely valuable, as did my own witnessing of events.

Because ACT UP was an ongoing movement at the time I did my interviews, my own methodology, although largely oral historical in nature, also incorporated a number of techniques more typical of ethnography.[9] As in ethnography, my research involved conducting interviews "in the context of ethnographic encounters involving large numbers of people"; I was able to analyze the behavior of activists as well as their words, and I engaged in an extended period of participant-observation work with both ACT UP chapters.[10] At the same time, my research methodology was distanced from ethnography in some crucial respects. First, in contrast to traditional ethnography, in which the recording of life histories and the experiencing of all aspects of the informants' lives is standard practice, my interest in my narrators was limited to their involvement with and knowledge of ACT UP, and the only context in which I witnessed most of my narrators was that of ACT UP–related events.[11] Second, although I was able to observe a period of the history of both ACT UP chapters, many of the events Rhode Island narrators described, and most of those described by New York activists, occurred long before my involvement with these groups. Finally, in contrast to standard anthropological practice, I never attempted to treat my experience of ACT UP as "cross-cultural."[12] Nonetheless, even though my methodology was primarily oral historical in nature, I found the opportunity to be involved with both ACT UP/RI and ACT UP/New York for a period of their respective histories invaluable when it came time to develop my own analysis.[13]

Because my interviews were conducted while ACT UP was an ongoing movement, I have referred to them in the past tense ("Craig remembered"), as opposed to the present tense references that are common in oral history ("Craig remembers"). While my interviews provide extensive evidence as to what ACT UP was like during the period from 1987-1993, they also demonstrate how certain activists felt about and remembered ACT UP at a particular moment in its history (1993), which may be considerably different from how these same activists felt about the group—and its past—in later years. In fact, although I considered interviewing more activists in 1996, I decided that it would be best not to "contaminate" the interviews from 1993 with recollections from a later year. Had ACT UP been a movement that had ended thirty years ago, I suspect that it would have been perfectly safe to interview activists in a number of different years. However, ACT UP was and still is an ongoing movement, and this has necessitated certain precautions, not the least of which is treating my narrators' statements as contingent to a particular historical moment.

Although the number of ACT UP members I was able to interview was only a small percentage of those who had been involved in each chapter, I attempted to make my interviews as representative as possible in a number of ways. I deliberately went out of my way to talk to current as well as former members, new members as well as those who had been involved for several years, women as well as men, people of color as well as white activists, and people involved with different committees. At the same time, because of the focus of my project, I also attempted to conduct as many interviews as possible with ACT UP members who were writers and with those activists who had been members of both ACT UP/New York and ACT UP/RI. For both ACT UP chapters, my interviews continued until I felt that activists were beginning to repeat one another.

Despite this level of intentionality in my choosing of narrators, in one respect I felt rather unrestricted in terms of my interview sampling: since I was not trying to construct a history of ACT UP, there were very few individual activists to whom I felt I absolutely had to speak. Although I did have the opportunity to talk to some of ACT UP's most prominent and outspoken members, I also made a deliberate attempt to interview people who had had a minimal role in ACT UP besides attending weekly meetings, who had recently joined the group, or who had left ACT UP after a brief involvement that was not to their liking. Because they were easier to locate, however, the majority of my narrators were involved with ACT UP at the time I did my interviewing.

Practitioners of oral history have disagreed about the appropriateness of editing interview transcripts in the direction of standard English. Since most people do not talk as eloquently as they write, some theorists have felt that replicating the spoken words of narrators verbatim has a tendency to make them look silly or unintelligent, thereby encouraging condescension on the part of readers.[14] My own approach to this problem is as follows. Quotes from activists in this study have been purged of verbal tics, such as "like" or "uh." More significantly, in places where the syntax of a speaker was garbled or confusing, I have cleaned it up just as much as was necessary to make the content of a statement clear. Where a statement was clear but not necessarily eloquent, however, I have kept it exactly as stated. Finally, as in written English, I have inserted ellipses wherever words or sentences have been removed from the middle of a quote.

Interviews were transcribed by me—a time-consuming task that stemmed to a considerable extent from lack of funds to hire an assistant, but which came with its own advantages as well. By transcribing the interviews myself, I was able to recall my conversations with activists and to experience their richness as spoken conversation much more fully and intimately than if I had simply been presented with pages of transcripts by an assistant. When it came time to turn these interviews into a narrative, the familiarity that the transcription process had afforded me seemed worth the extra time and effort.

The following is a list of the activists interviewed for this study. Although not all of them are quoted directly, all of the interviews proved invaluable in one way or another in the development of my analysis, and I am extremely grateful to the activists who took the time to provide them. Beside each name, I have indicated the ACT UP chapter(s) that each narrator reported having been affiliated with as of the time of the interview, in roughly the order joined (some affiliations were concurrent). The date of the interview is listed as well. Phone interviews are indicated with a (PH) next to the date; all other interviews were conducted in person. Cotter and Lee were interviewed together at their request, an arrangement that turned out to be extremely productive; all other interviews were one-on-one. Narrators were given the option at the time of the interview of using either their own name or a pseudonym of their choosing; names that are pseudonyms are indicated with quotation marks.

At the time I spoke with them, a number of narrators gave permission for their interviews to be shared with other scholars. However, although twenty-four narrators consented to have their interviews shared, I have decided to make only fifteen of these interviews available, both to protect the anonymity of those narrators who chose pseudonyms, and in order to respect the wishes of narrators who asked that particular statements be kept off the record. The interviews that are available are indicated with an asterisk next to the name of the narrator; the tapes can be found in the Special Collections Department of the Brown University Library, Providence, RI.

Name	ACT UP Affiliation	Date
Fred Adler	Rhode Island	April 22, 1993
Mary Cotter*	New York	July 27, 1993
B.C. Craig	Boston New York	July 7, 1993
Michael Cunningham	New York	October 3, 1993 (PH)
Kim Edwards	New York	July 13, 1993
David B. Feinberg*	New York	July 5, 1993
Kevin Robert Frost*	New York	August 19, 1993
Stephen Gendin*	New York Rhode Island	June 14, 1993
Keith Halperin	New York	August 11, 1993
Peter Hocking	Rhode Island	January 18, 1993
Joan Hofer*	Rhode Island	May 25, 1993
Bill Jesdale	Rhode Island	March 28, 1993
"Trina Johnson"	New York	June 15, 1993
"Travis Jones"	New York	August 14, 1993 (PH)
"Ann Kraft"	Rhode Island	March 14, 1993
Berna Lee*	New York	July 27, 1993
Carlos Maldonado	New York	August 12, 1993
James McGrath*	Rhode Island New York San Jose	April 4, 1993 (PH)
"Alan Petrofsky"	New York Rhode Island	May 11, 1993
M. Moore Robinson*	Washington, DC Rhode Island San Francisco	April 4, 1993 (PH)

Name	ACT UP Affiliation	Date
Mark Ruisi*	Rhode Island	January 21, 1993
Sarah Schulman	New York	July 20, 1993 (PH)
B.J. Sklar	Rhode Island	February 9, 1993
Duncan A. Smith*	Rhode Island	January 19, 1993
Norberto A. Stuart*	New York	July 2, 1993
Michael K. Swirsky*	New York	July 3, 1993
Jennifer Ting*	East Bay (CA) Rhode Island	March 10, 1993
John Weir*	New York	July 28, 1993
"Genine Whitlock"	Rhode Island	April 17, 1993 (PH)
Jon Winkleman*	Rhode Island New York	July 8, 1993
Maxine Wolfe	New York	August 4, 1993

Notes

Introduction

1. On ACT UP's tenth anniversary, see *POZ*, March 1997 (special issue on ACT UP).
2. Since my involvement with ACT UP/RI preceded my decision to study ACT UP by a number of years, my time with that group can only be considered fieldwork in retrospect.
3. For a more detailed theorization of my use of these interviews, see "Appendix: Research Methodology" in this book.
4. I am defining "politics" somewhat narrowly here; see my definition in the "Goals" section of Chapter 1.

Introduction to Part One

1. Jean-Christophe Agnew, "The Consuming Vision of Henry James," in *The Culture of Consumption: Critical Essays in American History, 1880-1980*, eds. Richard Wightman Fox and T.J. Jackson Lears (New York: Pantheon Books, 1983), p. 74.
2. Such an assertion, although definitely true for the period studied in these chapters, has recently been called into question by a new class of AIDS drugs called protease inhibitors. Although very expensive, they offer considerable hope for the people with AIDS (PWAs) who can in fact afford them. However, since no one has gone so far as to argue that protease inhibitors constitute a "cure" per se, I would still maintain that AIDS remains a crisis of consumption—even for the affluent, and even into the present.
3. On the ability of AIDS to "out" gay men, see Stephanie Bell, " 'Galpals' and 'Space Alien Drag Queens': Outing, AIDS, and Tabloid Newspapers," *Radical America* 25 (January-March 1991): 88-90; and Richard Meyer, "Rock Hudson's Body," in *Inside/Out: Lesbian Theories, Gay Theories,* ed. Diana Fuss (New York: Routledge, 1991), especially pp. 274-278. While it can probably go without saying that AIDS is not a "gay disease" it should be noted that AIDS is not a "disease," period. AIDS is a syndrome made up of a number of opportunistic infections (fungi, viruses, cancers, bacterial infections) that take advantage of the damage that an individual's immune system has incurred following infection with HIV. For many years, in fact, an AIDS diagnosis was dependent on the appearance of a certain threshold number of these opportunistic infections. People do not die from AIDS: they die

from the infections their immune system cannot fight off. This said, I will occasionally refer to AIDS as a "disease" in this study, largely as a form of shorthand. For a clarification of the differences between the terms "disease" and "syndrome" in relation to AIDS, see Jan Zita Grover, "AIDS: Keywords" in *AIDS: Cultural Analysis/ Cultural Activism*, ed. Douglas Crimp (Cambridge, MA: MIT Press, 1988), pp. 18-20.

4. Although my own background is in the interdisciplinary field of American studies, I am speaking here in general terms.

5. See, for instance, Lisa Duggan, "The Discipline Problem: Queer Theory Meets Lesbian and Gay History," *GLQ* 2 (1995, pp. 179-191), especially pp. 181 and 188; and Gayle Rubin with Judith Butler, "Sexual Traffic," *differences* 6 (Summer-Fall 1994):91-94.

6. I am indebted here to Diana Fuss. "The problem, of course, with the inside/ outside rhetoric, if it remains undeconstructed," Fuss writes, "is that such polemics disguise the fact that most of us are both inside and outside at the same time." Diana Fuss, *"Inside/Out,"* in Fuss, p. 5.

7. See Eric Rofes, *Reviving the Tribe: Regenerating Gay Men's Sexuality and Culture in the Ongoing Epidemic* (Binghamton, NY: Harrington Park Press, 1996).

8. Urvashi Vaid, *Virtual Equality: The Mainstreaming of Gay and Lesbian Liberation* (New York: Anchor Books, 1995), pp. 249-259. See also the essays in Part One of Amy Gluckman and Betsy Reed, eds., *Homo Economics: Capitalism, Community, and Lesbian and Gay Life* (New York: Routledge, 1997), many of which discuss the use and abuse of gay income statistics by the gay press, the mass media, and the right wing alike.

9. I am grateful to Sarah Schulman for reminding me of this fact during my interview with her.

10. Anthony Freitas, Susan Kaiser, and Tania Hammidi, "Communities, Commodities, Cultural Space, and Style," in *Gays, Lesbians, and Consumer Behavior: Theory, Practice, and Research Issues in Marketing*, ed. Daniel L. Wardlow (Binghamton, NY: Harrington Park Press, 1996), p. 89.

11. Nicola Field, *Over the Rainbow: Money, Class, and Homophobia* (London: Pluto Press, 1995), pp. 50-51.

Chapter 1

1. Presidential Debate Transcript, *The New York Times*, October 12, 1992:A17.

2. The brief history to ACT UP/New York that follows is drawn largely from "ACT UP/New York Capsule History," ACT UP/New York Web site (www.actupny.org); Douglas Crimp with Adam Rolston, *AIDS Demo Graphics*, (Seattle, WA: Bay Press, 1990); Maxine Wolfe, "The AIDS Coalition to Unleash Power (ACT UP): A Direct Model of Community Research for AIDS Prevention," in *AIDS Prevention and Services: Community Based Research*, ed. Johannes P. Van Vugt (Westport, CT: Bergin and Garvey, 1994); and the interviews I conducted with members. The introductory history to ACT UP/RI is based on both my own knowledge from working with the group and interviews with members. No comprehensive

history of ACT UP/New York exists, let alone one of ACT UP as a national movement, and my knowledge of ACT UP chapters outside of New York City and Providence, RI is limited. For a good snapshot of ACT UP as it existed nationwide in
1993 (the year that I did my fieldwork), see Sally Chew, "What's Going Down with
ACT UP?," *Out,* November 1993:72-75, 130-137.

   3. Larry Kramer, "The Beginning of ACTing UP," in *Reports from the
Holocaust: The Story of an AIDS Activist,* Updated and Expanded Edition (New
York: St. Martin's Press, 1994), p. 135. On some of the AIDS activism that laid
the groundwork for ACT UP, see Wolfe, "AIDS Coalition," pp. 217-220.

   4. For a discussion of some of the movements that did exist during this period,
see Barbara Epstein, *Political Protest and Cultural Revolution: Nonviolent Direct
Action in the 1970s and 1980s* (Berkeley: University of California Press, 1991).

   5. Although the exact makeup of ACT UP/New York is hard to establish and
shifted greatly over time, a survey conducted by Gilbert Elbaz in June and July of
1989 provides a more quantitative snapshot of the group than the qualitative discussion that follows. Elbaz reports that he received back 413 surveys out of the 450 that
he distributed. Of those responding, 79.7 percent self-identified as male; 78.5 percent
self-identified as white; 95 percent self-identified as having attended college or graduate school; 82.8 percent self-identified as professionals, white-collar workers, artists,
or students; one quarter self-identified as earning over $35,000 annually, and a little
less than 50 percent self-identified as earning $25,000-$35,000 annually; and only
5.1 percent self-identified as heterosexual. Gilbert Elbaz, "The Sociology of AIDS
Activism: The Case of ACT UP/New York, 1987-1992," (PhD dissertation, City
University of New York, 1992), pp. 65-69. While no such statistics exist for ACT
UP/RI, it is safe to say that the group had an even higher percentage of gay white
male members than did ACT UP/New York.

   6. It is important to stress here that there are many parts to, and versions of,
the story of ACT UP, only a few of which are discussed in this chapter. In particular, I have focused on the experiences of gay white men in the group, given that
my larger focus in this chapter is their experience of the epidemic. My analysis of
ACT UP is not intended to be the final word on the topic: a comprehensive history of the group has yet to be written.

   7. Such a description is at least somewhat applicable to many of the women
and people of color in ACT UP as well. As Travis Jones suggested, in fact, while
people-of-color caucuses in ACT UP/New York were often critical of ACT UP's frequent inability to recognize the AIDS-related needs of minority communities, "in
some ways, we [people of color] were as much out of touch with those communities
as were the people we were busy indicting." "If you looked at the Black Caucus,"
Jones noted, "most of us were coming to New York City from outside New York
City. Most of us, to the extent that we were black and poor, it was more historical
than it was current. We were probably somewhat closer to the level of ACT UP in
terms of education and socioeconomic status than we were with the minority community who was affected by AIDS." (Travis Jones, telephone interview.)

   8. By "unmarked," I mean dominant (and therefore invisible) in terms of
race and gender. (On the effect of AIDS on "unmarked" identities, see again the

Introduction to Part One of this book.) What I am suggesting here, in a way, is a cognitive theory of class privilege: certain individuals act entitled, get what they want (because they are white, or male, or middle class), and therefore continue to act this way in the future. In this way, class becomes a style—a way of acting—that produces predictable results, and thereby feeds (and normalizes) the sense of entitlement that produced it in the first place.

9. In addition to my own analysis of media coverage of ACT UP, see John Nguyet Erni, *Unstable Frontiers: Technomedicine and the Cultural Politics of "Curing" AIDS* (Minneapolis: University of Minnesota Press, 1994), pp. 96-99.

10. Gina Kolata, "Advocates' Tactics on AIDS Issues Provoking Warnings of a Backlash," *The New York Times*, March 11, 1990: sec. 4, p. 5; Bill Ervolino, "ACT UP Making Headlines—and Enemies," *The (Hackensack) Record*, February 10, 1993:A6; "The West Coast Gay Tantrum," editorial, *New York City Tribune*, June 22, 1990; "Civil Disobedience vs. Uncivilized Behavior," editorial, *New York Daily News*, December 12, 1989:28.

11. John Leo, "When Activism Becomes Gangsterism," *U.S. News and World Report*, February 5, 1990:18.

12. Ray Kerrison, column, *New York Post*, December 15, 1989:2.

13. Paula Span, "Getting Militant about AIDS: Vandalism, Confrontations Mark Escalating Protest," *Washington Post*, March 28, 1989:D1.

14. Randy Shilts, "Politics Confused with Therapy," *San Francisco Chronicle*, June 26, 1989:A4.

15. Richard D. Mohr, *Gay Ideas: Outing and Other Controversies* (Boston, MA: Beacon Press, 1992), pp. 275-276, n. 21.

16. Andrew Miller and Rex Wockner, "AIDS/Abortion Rights Demo Halts High Mass at St. Pat's," *OutWeek*, December 24, 1989:14.

17. Scott Craig, letter, *OutWeek*, January 14, 1990:7. For an opposing opinion from within the gay community, see "Over Whose Dead Bodies?" *OutWeek*, December 24, 1989:4. As Alan Petrofsky and Duncan A. Smith indicated in interviews with me, much of ACT UP/RI's local reputation as a "radical" organization stemmed from demonstrations organized by other ACT UP chapters, especially "Stop the Church."

18. Quotations from the original interviews I conducted as part of my fieldwork are not footnoted in this study. When either a quote from an activist or a statement attributed to an activist appears without a footnote, readers may assume that it is taken from these interviews. (Quotations from activists that are taken from previously published sources are, of course, footnoted.) The ACT UP chapter with which a narrator was affiliated is indicated in parenthesis following the narrator's name; if a narrator was a member of both ACT UP/New York and ACT UP/RI, both are indicated. Additional information on narrators is available in the Appendix.

19. Dave Ford, "A.I.D.S.: Words from the Front," *Spin*, January 1989:61.

20. For an overview of gay liberation thinking from the early 1970s, see Karla Jay and Allen Young, eds., *Out of the Closets: Voices of Gay Liberation*, Twentieth Anniversary Edition (New York: New York University Press, 1992).

21. Crimp with Rolston, *AIDS Demo Graphics*, p. 98.

22. Speech reprinted in "Duberman Addresses Stonewall Dedication," *Out-Week*, June 26,1989:20-21.

23. Carl Cohen, "Militant Morality: Civil Disobedience and Bioethics," *Hastings Center Report*, November/December 1989:23-25.

24. On the direct and indirect components of ACT UP's civil disobedience tradition, see Jon Carroll, "One White Guy Sittin' Around Rantin'," *San Francisco Chronicle*, July 3, 1991:E10; and Herbert R. Spiers, "AIDS and Civil Disobedience," *Hastings Center Report*, November/December 1989:34-35. B.C. Craig (NYC) and Stephen Gendin (NYC/RI) also discussed with me the indirect nature of much of ACT UP's civil disobedience. Interestingly, Gendin recalled that during ACT UP's "Seize the FDA" action in 1988, activists attempted to bridge the gap between direct and symbolic civil disobedience. "We weren't saying we were going to stop the FDA's actions," Gendin recalled. "It was like, 'We can do a better job than the FDA, so we're trying taking it over. We are trying to do what should be done.'"

25. Carroll, "One White Guy Sittin' Around Rantin'," p. E10.

26. See, for instance, Martin Luther King Jr.'s discussion of his critics in his famous "Letter from Birmingham City Jail" (Philadelphia: American Friends Service Committee, May 1963).

27. Alvin Novick, "Civil Disobedience in Time of AIDS," *Hastings Center Reports*, November/December 1989:36. See also Courtney S. Campbell, "Ethics and Militant AIDS Activism," in *AIDS and Ethics*, ed. Frederic G. Reamer (New York: Columbia University Press, 1991).

28. Joshua Gamson, "Silence, Death, and the Invisible Enemy: AIDS Activism and Social Movement 'Newness,'" in *Ethnography Unbound: Power and Resistance in the Modern Metropolis*, by Michael Burawoy, Alice Burton, Ann Arnett Ferguson, Kathryn J. Fox, Joshua Gamson, Nadine Gartrell, Leslie Hurst, Charles Kurzman, Leslie Salzinger, Josepha Schiffman, and Shiori Ui (Berkeley: University of California Press, 1991), p. 37.

29. Ibid., p. 38.

30. Alberto Melucci, John Keane, and Paul Mier, "New Perspectives on Social Movements: An Interview with Alberto Melucci," in Melucci, *Nomads of the Present: Social Movements and Individual Needs in Contemporary Society*, eds. John Keane and Paul Mier (Philadelphia, PA: Temple University Press, 1989), p. 219.

31. Melucci, Keane, and Mier, "New Perspectives," p. 222.

32. Melucci (Keane and Mier, eds.) *Nomads*, p. 12.

33. Alberto Melucci, "The Symbolic Challenge of Contemporary Movements," *Social Research* 52 (1985):812.

34. Melucci (Keane and Mier, eds.) *Nomads*, p. 23.

35. During kiss-ins, large groups of same-sex couples kissed on cue in public; die-ins revolved around a crowd of activists lying on the ground to simulate the thousands of Americans dead from AIDS; outing was the public declaration by activists of the homosexuality of closeted politicians and celebrities.

36. Although Gamson's article is based largely on a participant-observation study done with ACT UP/San Francisco, he also discusses other ACT UP chapters,

including ACT UP/New York. On the relation of New Social Movement theory to AIDS, see also Steven Epstein, *Impure Science: AIDS, Activism, and the Politics of Knowledge* (Berkeley: University of California Press, 1996), pp. 19-22.

37. Gamson, pp. 46-47.

38. Ibid., p. 37.

39. Ibid., pp. 48-50. Gamson begins his essay, for instance, by discussing ACT UP/New York's attendance at a New York Mets game at Shea stadium, during which activists displayed large banners with safe-sex messages targeted at heterosexual men.

40. Gamson, "Silence, Death, and the Invisible Enemy," p. 44.

41. See also Cindy Patton, *Inventing AIDS* (New York: Routledge, 1990), Chapter 6.

42. Maxine Wolfe distinguished for me "disciplined parties," in which members are required to follow the instructions of party leaders or face expulsion, and groups such as ACT UP that have no official hierarchy.

43. See Jim Hummel, "AIDS Activists Protest Bill of Rights Display," *Providence Journal,* October 21, 1990:B1, B11.

44. In its broadest sense, I understand "politics" to mean "contests over power, especially, but not exclusively, state power."

45. I am grateful to J.P. Gownder for assisting me in devising this formulation.

46. It is worth keeping in mind in this regard that drug production and testing, although under the purview of industry, is a process that is inseparable from government control: as we shall see, activists were particularly concerned early on with the effect that FDA regulations were having on the production of drugs by private pharmaceutical companies, and ACT UP worked with government regulatory agencies to create a number of policies that directly affected the drug production process (such as what became known as "parallel track testing," which allowed drug companies to release potentially effective drugs to individuals not eligible for specific trials).

47. In this regard, ACT UP's agenda was fairly consistent with that of the gay movement that had immediately preceded it. Although many of the lesbian and gay organizations that appeared immediately after the 1969 Stonewall riots had been largely liberationist in focus (the Gay Liberation Front and the Gay Activists Alliance are two of the best-known examples), these organizations were soon supplanted by more rights-focused groups (such as the National Gay Task Force), resulting in, as Robert Padgug and Gerald M. Oppenheimer note, "a community that had replaced human liberation with civil rights and equality as its major aims." See Robert A. Padgug and Gerald M. Oppenheimer, "Riding the Tiger: AIDS and the Gay Community," in *AIDS: The Making of a Chronic Disease,* eds. Elizabeth Fee and Daniel M. Fox (Berkeley: University of California Press, 1992), pp. 250-252.

48. Although ACT UP/New York members tended to travel across the country for demonstrations, local ACT UP chapters were more likely to participate in national demonstrations that were occurring in their own cities. Thus, ACT UP/DC

was a prominent participant in "Seize the FDA" and "Storm the NIH," while ACT UP/Atlanta was highly involved in ACT UP demonstrations directed against the CDC.

49. *Voices from the Front,* videotape. Produced by Testing the Limits Collective, 1991.

50. Peter Staley, interview in *Voices from the Front.*

51. Crimp with Rolston, *AIDS Demo Graphics,* p. 79.

52. Crimp with Rolston, *AIDS Demo Graphics,* pp. 76-83; *Voices from the Front.*

53. *Voices from the Front;* Cliff O'Neil, "Demonstrators Rain Fire and Brimstone on NIH Headquarters," *OutWeek,* June 6, 1990:14-16.

54. *Voices from the Front;* O'Neil, "Demonstrators Rain Fire," pp. 14-16; Mark Harrington, "Let My People In," *OutWeek,* August 8, 1990:34. People of color were often excluded from government-sponsored drug trials on the grounds that they purportedly did not make reliable research subjects, and women were prohibited from entering trials out of concern that if they became pregnant, the drug being tested might damage the fetus.

55. Nina Reyes, "Hundreds of Women Storm CDC over AIDS Definition," *OutWeek,* December 19, 1990:16-17; Wolfe, "AIDS Coalition," pp. 233-234; Gena Corea, *The Invisible Epidemic: The Story of Women and AIDS* (New York: Harper-Collins, 1992), pp. 259-269; Elbaz, "The Sociology of AIDS Activism," pp. 177-182; Cindy Patton, *Last Served?: Gendering the HIV Pandemic* (London: Taylor and Francis, 1994), p. 86; and Maxine Wolfe, unpublished manuscript, pp. 41-43. (I am grateful to Maxine Wolfe for allowing me to use unpublished sections of what would eventually become her essay "AIDS Coalition.")

56. In addition to government agencies, ACT UP was willing (even eager) to work with other existing institutions with dubious ideological credentials in order to promote its agenda. For instance, many ACT UP members viewed the American media as a blank slate that could be put to use by activists, rather than as a tool of the dominant classes that would have to be either eliminated or worked around. What ACT UP did, Stephen Gendin (NYC/RI) explained, was "still based upon the idea that what the media does is use people, so rather than it being them using us, let's [have it be] us using them. As opposed to, let's create a media that really is for the people and that's truthful and honest." As such, Gendin argued, ACT UP demonstrated a strategy of "turn the system against itself," rather than a desire to replace the system with something better.

57. Bruce Nussbaum, *Good Intentions: How Big Business and the Medical Establishment Are Corrupting the Fight Against AIDS, Alzheimer's, Cancer, and More* (New York: Penguin, 1991), p. 290.

58. Philip M. Kayal, *Bearing Witness: Gay Men's Health Crisis and the Politics of AIDS* (Boulder, CO: Westview Press, 1993), p. 92.

59. Ibid., p. 91.

60. Richard Mohr for one has been a harsh critic of ACT UP's commitment to state intervention concerning AIDS, which he has viewed as inconsistent with ACT UP's overall critique of government intrusions into the rights of PWAs. "I hope

that ACT UP and others involved in AIDS funding and welfare issues will realize," Mohr points out, "that, although they may be protesting the state here and
there, at the molar level they are worshipping the state. Government funds never
come without strings—as we know from government funding of safe-sex literature." Mohr, *Gay Ideas,* pp. 52-53. The question of how much oppressed groups
should rely on the state for protection or services has been one that has troubled a
number of progressive theorists as well, especially when the state itself has been
a major source of grievance. See, for instance, Wendy Brown, "Finding the Man in
the State," *Feminist Studies* 18 (Spring 1992); Kimberlé Williams Crenshaw, "Race,
Reform, and Retrenchment: Transformation and Legitimation in Antidiscrimination
Law," *Harvard Law Review* 101 (May 1988):1366-1369; and Nan D. Hunter, "Marriage, Law, and Gender: A Feminist Inquiry," *Law and Sexuality: A Review of
Lesbian and Gay Legal Issues* 1 (Summer 1991):27-30.

61. As Wolfe notes, both condom-distribution and needle-exchange work within
ACT UP occupied the difficult position of "straddling the line between traditional
concepts of 'service' and 'action.'" Wolfe, unpublished manuscript, p. 48.

62. Ibid., pp. 43-48.

63. Ibid., pp. 48-54.

64. Ibid., p. 44. The quote appears in Wolfe's essay but is unattributed.

65. In 1993, ACT UP/New York mobilized in coalition with other organizations against the largest instance of HIV-related quarantine in U.S. history—the
internment of almost 300 Haitian refugees in Guantanamo Bay, Cuba. Denied
entry to the United States (despite their approved refugee status) because of U.S.
policy banning the permanent entry of foreigners with HIV, HIV-positive refugees
and their family members were kept in dangerously substandard internment camps
for over a year until a judicial ruling forced their release in 1993. See "Haitians with
HIV Are Being Murdered in a U.S. Military Concentration Camp," ACT UP/New
York document, 1993, ACT UP/New York archives.

66. Patton contrasts what she believes to be the position of gays as distinct
minorities with that of drug users, whom she argues were understood within the
category "addict," "a partial and highly pathologized identity which could succeed
only in pressing for more *treatment,* and not for civil and political rights for drug
users. Claims for these rights would come to the extent that drug users were
members of ethnic or racial groups already identified under civil rights rhetoric."
Patton, *Inventing AIDS,* p. 139, n. 24.

67. The fact that both ACT UP/New York and ACT UP/RI functioned along a
system of majority rule is crucial here, since it allowed the class style and the political priorities of white, middle-class gay men to come to dominate the organization.
When I asked Berna Lee (NYC) why she repeatedly referred to ACT UP as a group
of all white men during our interview when women and people of color formed an
important presence, Lee, a Korean American, responded, "A lot of the agenda is set
by issues that concern white men. . . . That's the majority of it, and when you have a
democracy, the majority rules."

Other ACT UP chapters, such as ACT UP/San Francisco, operated under a
system of consensus, which gave minority voices considerably more weight in the

decision-making process. It is interesting to note, however, that in September 1990, a group of mostly white men split off from ACT UP/San Francisco to form ACT UP/Golden Gate, in part because of concern over ACT UP/San Francisco's consensus system, and in part because of a feeling that some members of the group were assigning more importance to fighting racism, sexism, and other structural oppressions than to working for a cure. See Rachel Pepper, "Schism Slices ACT UP in Two," *OutWeek,* October 10, 1990:12-14.

68. On the relative politicization of men and women in ACT UP, see Elbaz, "The Sociology of AIDS Activism," pp. 76-82. Elbaz bases his analysis on a survey he conducted in 1989 and on interviews. His results confirm the more impressionistic evidence I gathered while interviewing activists in 1993.

The story of Peter Staley's transformation from a conservative Wall Street trader to a full-time ACT UP activist is frequently cited as the paradigmatic example of the politicization of men in the group. See "United in Anger," *NYQ,* December 8, 1991:29; and Elinor Burkett, *The Gravest Show on Earth: America in the Age of AIDS* (Boston: Houghton Mifflin, 1995), Chapter 12.

69. Ford, "A.I.D.S.: Words from the Front," p. 60.

70. Elbaz, "The Sociology of AIDS Activism," p. 77.

71. Maxine Wolfe, personal interview. See also "The AIDS Movement and Its Challenge," *Radical America* 21 (November/December 1988):62.

72. This conflict was somewhat reductively known as the "treatment versus social issues" or "treatment versus access" debate. One early example of ACT UP/New York's incorporating such a critique into its activist platform occurred during the September 1989 demonstration against Burroughs Wellcome, the makers of AZT, at which ACT UP called for "free AZT." See Crimp with Rolston, *AIDS Demo Graphics,* pp. 114-119.

73. As I wrote in a flyer for a Rhode Island demonstration on this issue, under a new federal AIDS definition that went into effect in 1992, persons with CD4+ (or T-cell) counts below 200 are now considered to have AIDS, even if they are not otherwise sick (in lay terms, CD4+ cells are a building block of the immune system: the fewer one has, the weaker his or her immune system). ACT UP chapters objected not so much to this new definition as to the requirement that the labs doing CD4+ testing should send the names of people with low CD4+ counts directly to the state departments of health; activists argued that people with HIV were having their CD4+ counts checked for their own information, not that of health officials, and that the health departments should maintain their previous policy of having all diagnosis information come exclusively from physicians' offices. ACT UP/New York did organizing concerning this and other testing issues as well, but such efforts generally took a backseat to organizing around treatments and a cure.

74. As Swirsky noted as well, organizing concerning privacy and other civil liberties concerns was also of key importance in states "where HIV tests are used to discriminate, those that basically have laws that essentially criminalize HIV status" (in 1993, for instance, Colorado and Michigan had statutes criminalizing con-

sensual sexual activity by HIV-positive individuals unless they informed their partners of their status, even if safer sex was practiced).

75. Bill Jesdale (ACT UP/RI), personal interview.

76. An ACT UP/RI flyer I helped to write explains concisely the difference between anonymous and confidential HIV testing: "With anonymous testing, you never have to give your name or other identifying information at the testing site. With confidential testing, your name is kept in a medical record that includes your test results. Because anonymous testing provides better privacy (and therefore better protection against discrimination), ACT UP/RI [among other chapters] has long endorsed it over confidential testing." ACT UP/RI document, 1993, photocopy. On ACT UP/RI's work on these issues, see also Lisa Prevost, "ACT UP Leery of Reduction in Anonymous HIV Testing Sites," *Newpaper* (Providence), April 4, 1991:2; and Felice J. Freyer, "ACT-UP Rallies Against AIDS Tracking Policy," *Providence Journal Bulletin,* October 21, 1993:D17.

77. Maxine Wolfe, personal interview; Kevin Robert Frost, personal interview; Wolfe, unpublished manuscript, p. 62. I use the terms "inside" and "outside" throughout this section because these are the terms with which activists themselves described their differing tactical approaches both in print and during my interviews with them. For further discussion of this tendency, see the Appendix.

78. The phrase "a place at the table" has had particular resonance for discussions of gay politics following the 1993 publication of Bruce Bawer's controversial *A Place at the Table: The Gay Individual in American Society* (New York: Poseidon, 1993).

79. B.C. Craig, personal interview; Cathy Jean Cohen, "Power, Resistance and the Construction of Crisis: Marginalized Communities Respond to AIDS," (PhD dissertation, University of Michigan, 1993), p. 314.

80. Maxine Wolfe suggested to me after reading an earlier version of this chapter that the history of ACT UP/New York can be divided into three periods, which I would date as follows: an early period running roughly from 1987-1989, a middle period running from 1989-1991, and a later period beginning around 1992, during which the McClintock Project was developed. In Wolfe's opinion, the ascendancy of a middle-class "class style" that I describe in this chapter is best located in the middle period, during which ACT UP changed both its mode of fund-raising and many of its priorities, as well as experienced its greatest growth. Prior to this period, ACT UP's relative lack of resources and access gave it a more traditional grassroots flavor; and as I will discuss, the departure of a number of key treatment activists in 1991 and 1992 represented a substantial milestone for the group as well. I am not entirely sure whether I agree with Wolfe's assessment here: much of the evidence in this chapter suggests that a middle-class "class style" was evident in one form or another throughout ACT UP's history. Still, Wolfe's observation should remind us that ACT UP/New York was (and still is) a constantly evolving organization, one whose goals and tactics shifted considerably over time.

81. George M. Carter, *ACT UP, the AIDS War, and Activism,* Pamphlet Series, no. 15 (Westfield, NJ: Open Magazine, 1992), p. 2.

82. Mark Golden, "ACT UP Redux," *QW*, October 11, 1992:22-25. Golden's respondents did express concern about the dangers of working too closely with government officials, a concern I will address at length shortly.

83. Wolfe, "AIDS Coalition," pp. 226-230; Crimp with Rolston, *AIDS Demo Graphics*, pp. 76-83.

84. Nina Reyes, "ACT UP T and D Plans Spinoff," *NYQ*, November 24, 1991:9; Burkett, *The Gravest Show on Earth*, pp. 333-341. TAG began as an affinity group of ACT UP, but eventually broke all ties with the larger group.

85. ACT UP/RI had a curious habit of using the term "subcommittee" for what most organizations would describe as a "committee." ACT UP/RI had no "committees"—any subgrouping of activists that did work outside of the general Tuesday night meetings was known as a "subcommittee."

86. DeBuono would later become the Health Commissioner for the State of New York .

87. Maxine Wolfe, personal interview; Kevin Robert Frost, personal interview; Wolfe, unpublished manuscript, p. 62.

88. The election of Bill Clinton in 1992 might also have had something to do with the decline of street activism around the time I did my fieldwork. Many activists viewed Clinton as more sympathetic to AIDS issues than Presidents Reagan or Bush and modified their activism accordingly, although much of the enthusiasm for Clinton had worn off by the summer of 1993, when I conducted my fieldwork. "Suddenly," Sarah Schulman (NYC) noted, "it was just like, 'Oh, we're in the White House now, blah blah blah,' and groups like ACT UP really didn't know how obstructive or oppositional to be, because it was unclear what was going to happen." Sarah Schulman, telephone interview.

89. As Gendin noted, although ACT UP/RI engaged in only one action in which arrests occurred, it organized other demonstrations and zaps in which arrest, although not a desired goal of the action, was a distinct possibility. Throughout its history, moreover, ACT UP/RI members also engaged in illegal activities of a more furtive nature, such as wheat pasting posters onto public property and other acts of minor vandalism (see my earlier discussion of ACT UP/RI's "art projects").

90. Cathy Cohen, "Power, Resistance and the Construction of Crisis," p. 314.

91. Wolfe, "AIDS Coalition," p. 234.

92. Corea, *The Invisible Epidemic*, pp. 224-225.

93. Harrington, "Let My People In," p. 34.

94. Linda Meredith, letter, *OutWeek*, August 22, 1990:5.

95. Tracy D. Morgan, letter, *OutWeek*, August 22, 1990:6.

96. Peter Staley, "Has the Direct-Action Group ACT UP Gone Astray?" *Advocate*, July 30, 1991:98.

97. Mark Harrington, "A Fifth Anniversary Letter to ACT UP," March 9, 1992, ACT UP/New York archives. It is worth noting that, although most activists cited in this section described themselves as being in favor of a joint inside/outside approach, several have been openly accused of advocating one over the other. Harrington's "Open Letter," for instance, accused Wolfe of pushing exclusively for an outside approach (a charge that Wolfe denies), while, as Morgan's letter suggests, Harrington

himself was frequently identified with an excessive commitment to inside channels. On the one hand, such a discrepancy could be indicative of the extent to which activist rhetoric had consolidated around a party line: although activists were likely to claim that they favored an "inside/outside" strategy, they clearly had different interpretations of what exactly such a strategy entailed. On the other hand, it is worth keeping in mind that such a discrepancy could point to the ways in which relatively minor differences in opinion can be interpreted as major disagreements within the context of an organization in which people's politics are necessarily close.

98. Ibid. The quote is unattributed.

99. Wolfe, unpublished manuscript, pp. 65-67. The moratorium proposal failed.

100. *Voices from the Front.*

101. Not all ACT UP members I spoke to shared these opinions, however. "I understand their point," Frost (NYC) noted, "and I think it's a valid point in the sense that we have to constantly guard against getting so cozy that we can't do an action, or we can't be highly critical. But I don't think from my perspective that has ever been the case. . . . I don't think anybody said, 'Oh, let's not go after Fauci, I actually like him.' "

102. Mary Lou DeCiantis was the Chief Administrator of the Office of AIDS/STD, Rhode Island Department of Health.

103. In a 1993 article in *Out* magazine examining the rising sentiment that ACT UP was on the decline, Sally Chew argued that the benefits of insider access perhaps outweighed the attendant lack of publicity for the organization. "There has arguably been some loss to the public," she noted, "—less information going out and fewer recruits coming in—but the gains on the inside have been considerable, thanks in part to the threat of direct action." Chew, "What's Going Down with ACT UP?," p. 131.

104. Wolfe "AIDS Coalition," p. 244, n. 18.

105. Elbaz, "The Sociology of AIDS Activism," pp. 481-482.

106. B.C. Craig, personal interview.

107. On the AIDS Conference expenditures, see Burkett, *The Gravest Show on Earth*, pp. 317-318. Except for the expenses associated with the conference, all amounts listed here are 1993 figures from budget documents distributed at meetings.

108. I've chosen to discuss this particular crisis because it occurred during the time I spent with ACT UP/New York in the summer of 1993. As such, I was able to follow the crisis closely, as well as to attend a number of emergency finance meetings that were held in its wake.

109. "ACT UP Treasury Report January 1, 1993-June 1, 1993," photocopy.

110. Both the collapse of the art market in the early 1990s and the fact that no one had the time or energy to organize a fund-raising event of a similar scale meant that the kinds of money that the famed art auctions had pumped into ACT UP in 1989 and 1990 were no longer available.

111. Sitting in on the weekly ACT UP meetings in which this growing financial crisis was discussed, I was astonished (as were a number of other activists) to witness the amount of denial that accompanied the crisis. Individuals and committees continued to request approval of large expenditures from the group, forc-

ing other activists to remind people over and over again that ACT UP simply had no money. At one meeting, an activist stood up and reminded the floor that if GMHC operated with the kind of financial mismanagement that ACT UP had recently fallen into, ACT UP would organize a demonstration.

112. B.C. Craig, who had an extensive history of involvement in previous activist movements, commented on the way such a reliance on money distanced ACT UP from its predecessors. ACT UP's approach to activism, according to Craig, "teaches people a lot about activism is money, and without money you can't be a good activist. Whereas people have been fighting for years out of their living rooms with stolen Xerox and magic marker signs. We [ACT UP] would never dream of doing such a thing!"

113. On the exceptionality of uprisings among the poor, see Frances Fox Piven and Richard A. Cloward, *Poor People's Movements: Why They Succeed, How They Fail* (New York: Vintage, 1979), pp. 6-14. Cathy Cohen offers an extension of this paradigm to the AIDS movement itself. See Cathy Cohen, "Power, Resistance and the Construction of Crisis," pp. 481-482.

114. For an excellent discussion of the purported "decline" of ACT UP chapters nationwide during this period, see Chew, "What's Going Down with ACT UP?". Chew's piece reads as a rebuttal to ACT UP naysayers who had been overly quick to point to the group's decline, while my analysis concentrates in greater detail on individual members' feelings about what had gone wrong. For another look at this transition period, see "Battle Fatigue," *The New Yorker,* November 9, 1992:39-40.

115. In referring to a shrinking membership and involvement here, I am thinking primarily of a decrease in participation on the part of members who had at one point been very active in the organization. ACT UP/New York also experienced a more notable (although perhaps fundamentally less significant) exit on the part of a large number of individuals who were drawn to ACT UP because it was fashionable but whose actual involvement beyond attending meetings was slight.

116. This section will focus on ACT UP/New York to the exclusion of ACT UP/RI. Although ACT UP/RI endorsed initiatives such as universal health care and the McClintock Project, these radical responses to ACT UP's malaise were spearheaded by ACT UP chapters that had a history of focusing on issues of national concern. ACT UP/RI's response to its own sense of decline was somewhat different from the developments I am about to describe: primarily frustrated by its movement from the street to the conference table (a move that a small group such as ACT UP/RI found extremely difficult to pull off), ACT UP/RI returned to the street with major demonstrations in October and December 1993. The following year, ACT UP/RI made something of a return to its early tactic of "Art Projects," by focusing most of its energies on a campaign in which first-person narratives about living with AIDS were postered around Providence. On the demonstrations, see Freyer, "ACT-UP Rallies Against AIDS Tracking Policy"; and Jody McPhillips, "ACT UP! Protests at Journal," *Providence Journal Bulletin,* December 16, 1993, D19.

117. Such grief found political outlets occasionally, including a series of funerals in which the ashes or even bodies of deceased members were carried through Washington to symbolize government inaction—and, more important, to allow for a genu-

ine mourning process. See Simon Watney, "Political Funeral," *Village Voice*, October 20, 1992:18; and Frederic M. Biddle, "ACT UP's Last Act?" *Boston Globe Magazine*, September 5, 1993:13, 25-28. (Biddle's article also discusses the difficulties that affected chapters nationwide.)

118. Except where otherwise noted, all information about the content of this project comes from ACT UP/New York's booklet *The Barbara McClintock Project to Cure AIDS*, thousands of copies of which were distributed nationwide. (The document can also be found on the ACT UP/New York Web site, www.actupny.org.) Activists declined the use of the name "Manhattan Project" in order to distance their proposed research effort from a project that resulted in the creation of weapons of mass destruction. The project was eventually renamed "The AIDS Cure Project."

119. B.C. Craig, personal interview; Kevin Robert Frost, personal interview.

120. Elbaz, "The Sociology of AIDS Activism," pp. 442-467.

121. Jacob Smith Yang, "Activists Protest Inside Capital," *Gay Community News*, October 6-12, 1991, pp. 3, 6. The ACT UP/Network prepared a handbook to accompany the demonstration. See ACT UP/Network, *Universal Health Care: A Handbook for Activists* (Los Angeles, CA: ACT UP/Network, 1991).

122. Tony Arn and Gunther Freehill, "Demanding Universal Health Care," in *Universal Health Care*, p. 3.

123. On the October 1991 demonstration and the 1992 presidential campaign, see Elbaz, "The Sociology of AIDS Activism," pp. 467-470. A single payer system (similar to that in Canada) would have replaced insurance companies with one health care payer—the government. During the recent debates on national health care, more moderate factions (such as the Clinton Administration itself) proposed plans allowing for the continued existence of health insurance companies. See Norman Daniels, *Seeking Fair Treatment: From the AIDS Epidemic to National Health Care Reform* (New York: Oxford University Press, 1995), pp. 156-157.

Chapter 2

1. Paul Monette's best-known works are actually two of his nonfiction pieces: *Borrowed Time: An AIDS Memoir* (New York: Harcourt Brace Jovanovich, 1988) and *Becoming a Man: Half a Life Story* (New York: Harcourt Brace Jovanovich, 1992). For an overview of Monette's literary career, see David Román, "Paul Monette," in *Contemporary Gay American Novelists: A Bio-Bibliographical Critical Sourcebook*, ed. Emmanuel S. Nelson (Westport, CT: Greenwood Press, 1993), pp. 272-281. Monette died of complications from AIDS in 1995.

2. See Monette, *Borrowed Time*.

3. Paul Monette, personal correspondence, October 13, 1993. On the *Thirtysomething* episode, see Maria Maggenti, "No Half Measures" (interview with Paul Monette), *OutWeek*, May 8, 1991:56. For Monette's description of his attitudes toward and work with ACT UP and other political organizations, see the essays in *Last Watch of the Night: Essays Too Personal and Otherwise* (New York: Harcourt Brace and Company, 1994), especially "Mustering," "Getting Covered," and "Puck." A group closely resembling ACT UP makes a cameo appearance in *Afterlife*.

4. Paul Monette, *Afterlife* (New York: Crown Publishers, Inc., 1990), p. 222. All further references will appear in the body of the text.

5. As Jean Baudrillard has written, "The whole discourse on consumption, whether learned or lay, is articulated on the mythological sequence of the fable: a man, 'endowed' with needs which 'direct' him towards objects that 'give' him satisfaction. Since man is really never satisfied . . . the same history is repeated indefinitely." Jean Baudrillard, "Consumer Society," in *Selected Writings*, ed. Mark Poster (Stanford, CA: Stanford University Press, 1988), p. 35. For a historical approach to the built-in limits of consumption, see the introduction to Richard Wightman Fox and T.J. Jackson Lears, *The Culture of Consumption: Critical Essays in American History, 1880-1980* (New York: Pantheon Books, 1983), especially pp. vii-xii.

6. Sonny fails to learn this lesson, continuing to evaluate lovers based on their wealth. Sonny is evocatively described early in *Afterlife* as being "in the market again" (p. 6), and his search for a lover ends in degradation and defeat as Sean Pfieffer cuts off their short romance, giving a shocked Sonny an envelope containing $2,000. Sonny reaps what he has sown, of course—in viewing potential lovers in terms of their spending power (a process Mark and Steven increasingly eschew), Sonny sets himself up to find the tables turned, his hopes for a permanent relationship reduced to a cash settlement.

7. As Marx points out in *Capital,* commodity fetishism is a process in which imagined relationships between objects (commodities) come to occlude the real social relationships that exist between people (their producers), and in which commodities are invested with lives of their own. Thus, in abandoning commodities for human relations, Mark and Steven reverse this fetishistic process. See Karl Marx, *Capital: A Critique of Political Economy*, vol. 1 (1887; New York, International Publishers, 1967), pp. 71-83; and David Harvey, *The Condition of Postmodernity: An Enquiry into the Origins of Cultural Change* (Cambridge, MA: Blackwell, 1990), pp. 100-101. On the "transcendent" nature of the commodity, see Marx, *Capital*, p. 71.

8. In a related argument, John Clum has discussed the nostalgic remembrance by older gay writers of an affluent, carefree, pre-AIDS existence. His argument includes a discussion of Monette's poetry, as well as some of the other AIDS-related texts in which consumption and commodities play a central role. See John Clum, "'And Once I Had It All': AIDS Narratives and Memories of an American Dream," in *Writing AIDS: Gay Literature, Language, and Analysis*, eds. Timothy F. Murphy and Suzanne Poirier (New York: Columbia University Press, 1993), pp. 200-224.

9. For a good overview of Kramer's political and artistic career, see "Larry Kramer," *Current Biography*, March 1994:20-24.

10. See Kramer, *Reports from the Holocaust: The Story of an AIDS Activist,* Updated and Expanded Edition (New York: St. Martin's Press, 1994), pp. 30-32. For nonfictional accounts of Kramer's tumultuous involvement with GMHC, see also the other essays in that volume, especially the pieces dating from 1981-1983. Other accounts of this involvement include Bruce Nussbaum, *Good Intentions: How Big Business and the Medical Establishment Are Corrupting the Fight Against AIDS, Alzheimer's, Cancer, and More* (New York: Penguin, 1991), pp. 103-107, and

Randy Shilts, *And the Band Played On: Politics, People, and the AIDS Epidemic* (New York: Penguin, 1988), Chapters 12-30.

11. See, for instance, Larry Kramer, "An Open Letter to Richard Dunne and Gay Men's Health Crisis," in Kramer, *Reports,* p. 109.

12. Although the organization that Ned Weeks helps to found is never given a name, Kramer's own role in the formation of GMHC makes it the obvious candidate. The action in the play does roughly correspond with Kramer's own experiences with GMHC, and commentators have been able to draw connections between the characters in the play and actual individuals. (For example, Dinitia Smith identifies the characters Bruce, Mickey, and Tommy as GMHC founders Paul Popham, Larry Mass, and Rodger McFarlane, respectively. Dinitia Smith, "The Cry of 'The Normal Heart,'" *New York,* June 3, 1985:46.) As I will discuss in Chapter 3, however, it is crucial to remember that Kramer's depiction of GMHC in *The Normal Heart,* although grounded in his own experiences, is ultimately an imaginative rather than a historical one. As such, I will refer to it simply as "the AIDS organization" in my analysis.

13. Kramer, *Reports,* p. 94.

14. Kramer, *Reports,* p. 213. See also Kramer's comments in L.A. Winokur, "I Was Not a Political Animal Before AIDS" (interview with Larry Kramer), *The Progressive,* June 1994:32-35.

15. Kramer, *Reports,* p. xxxii.

16. Larry Kramer, *The Normal Heart* (New York: Plume, 1985), p. 45. All further references will appear in the body of the text.

17. Ben's economic privilege is most directly symbolized by the two-million-dollar house he plans to build for his family, a model of which is actually rolled onto the stage in Scene 6. Even Ned objects to such expenditure, but only because his AIDS organization is so underfunded by the city. When Felix appears in Scene 5 with an eighteen-dollar pint of gourmet ice cream, Ned demonstrates no such objections to conspicuous consumption.

18. For an extensive discussion of Kramer's endorsement of activism at the end of *The Normal Heart,* see Chapter 3.

19. Schulman's career as an activist both preceded and extended beyond her involvement with ACT UP. In 1992, in fact, Schulman cofounded the Lesbian Avengers, a lesbian direct action organization that she herself has described as having "established a new tone for lesbian politics—a post-ACT UP lesbian movement." See Schulman, "The Lesbian Avengers, Part One," in *My American History: Lesbian and Gay Life During the Reagan/Bush Years* (New York: Routledge, 1994), p. 282. On Schulman's involvement with and thinking about ACT UP/ New York, see also the other essays in the collection, especially "Preface: My Life as an American Artist," "Introduction," "Delusions of Gender," "Whatever Happened to Lesbian Activism," and "The Denial of AIDS and the Construction of a Fake Life."

20. "I came in very suspicious," Schulman noted in my interview with her in reference to her joining a male-dominated movement such as ACT UP. "You

know, I had never worked with gay men before; I had had the whole experience with the pre-AIDS movement, where gay men just wanted to access the same privileges as straight men." Sarah Schulman, telephone interview.

21. Schulman's novels include *The Sophie Horowitz Story* (Tallahassee, FL: Naiad, 1984), *Girls, Visions, and Everything* (Seattle, WA: Seal Press, 1986), *After Delores* (New York: Dutton, 1988), *People in Trouble* (New York: Dutton, 1990), *Empathy* (New York: Dutton, 1992), and *Rat Bohemia* (New York: Dutton, 1995). Many of the essays she has written for the gay, feminist, and progressive press are collected in *My American History*.

22. Sarah Schulman, "My Life as an American Artist," in *My American History*, pp. xviii-xix. For further discussion of the impediments faced by openly lesbian writers in the literary marketplace, see Schulman's essay "Is Lesbian Culture Only For Beginners?" in the same volume, as well as her afterword to that essay.

23. Sarah Schulman, phone interview. "I wanted a book that was accusatory to straight people for their abandonment of us," she noted. (All remaining quotes from Schulman that are not footnoted are taken from my interview with her.)

24. Sarah Schulman, *People in Trouble* (New York: Dutton, 1990), p. 66. All further references will appear in the body of the text.

25. Quoted in Andrea Freud Loewenstein, "Troubled Times" (interview with Sarah Schulman), *Women's Review of Books*, July 1990:23.

26. One is reminded here of television movies about AIDS that are primarily concerned with how the epidemic affects the family of the PWA, rather than the PWA him- or herself, a move which manages to position the family as the ultimate "victim" of the epidemic. See Paula A. Treichler, "AIDS Narratives on Television: Whose Story?" in Murphy and Poirier, *Writing AIDS*, pp. 161-199. Schulman herself makes reference to this phenomenon on page 73 of *People in Trouble*.

27. Sarah Schulman, telephone interview. As Steven F. Kruger has noted, by depicting Horne in an unmistakably satiric manner, Schulman is able to signal that he represents "a particular constellation of capitalist enterprise, political ambition, racist, sexist, and homophobic animus," thereby distancing her novel from others that view AIDS as the intentional doing of individual villains. Horne is not a villain per se, but "a figure for a whole matrix of (economic, political, societal) processes lying beyond the intentional control of any one individual." Kruger, *AIDS Narratives: Gender and Sexuality, Fiction and Science* (New York: Garland, 1996), p. 267.

28. Ironically enough, as Schulman herself noted, "by the time the book was published," ACT UP "had already gone beyond what I was proposing" in several respects. For instance, although *People in Trouble* depicts a demonstration at St. Patrick's Cathedral involving forty silent protesters, 5,000 angry demonstrators would eventually attend ACT UP's "Stop the Church" demonstration in December 1989.

29. Sarah Schulman, "Thousands May Die in the Streets: AIDS and the Homeless," in *My American History*, pp. 180-184.

Chapter 3

1. Paul Monette, *Afterlife* (New York: Crown Publishers, Inc., 1990), p. 173.

2. See, for instance, the introduction to Therese Jones, ed., *Sharing the Delirium: Second Generation AIDS Plays and Performances* (Portsmouth, NH: Heinemann, 1994).

3. The world premiere of *Millennium Approaches* (the first half of *Angels in America*) took place in 1991, and that of *Perestroika* (the second half) occurred in 1992, although rewrites of *Perestroika* continued into 1993. The published versions of Tony Kushner's *Millennium Approaches* (New York: Theatre Communications Group, 1993) and *Perestroika* (New York: Theatre Communications Group, 1994) contain useful chronologies of their respective production histories.

4. Kushner's commitment to building a wide audience can be most closely traced to his decision to move the New York premier of *Angels in America* from the Public Theater to the Walter Kerr on Broadway. See Bruce Weber, "*Angels'* Angels," *The New York Times Magazine,* April 25, 1993:29-30, 48-58; and Bruce Weber, "'Angels,' Downtown or on Broadway?" *The New York Times,* November 13, 1992:C2. Kramer has discussed his desire for a broad (and, he implies, heterosexual) audience for *The Normal Heart* in his own writings. See Larry Kramer, *Reports from the Holocaust: The Story of an AIDS Activist,* Updated and Expanded Edition (New York: St. Martin's Press, 1994), p. 94. Both men got their wishes: *Angels* won the approval of the mainstream theater establishment through its winning of the Pulitzer Prize for drama in 1993 and two Tony Awards for Best Play (one for each half), and *The Normal Heart* has been seen in hundreds of productions around the country and the world.

5. On the somewhat narrow definition of "politics" that informs my analysis here, see again the "Goals" section of Chapter 1. The term "politics plot" in this chapter is used as a parallel to "love plot." What I mean by it is not a plot that is political (which all plots are), but a plot that is specifically concerned on the level of content with the activities of politicians, activists, and/or government players. The seminal work on novels containing such plots is undoubtedly Irving Howe, *Politics and the Novel* (1957; New York: Columbia University Press, 1992). For two good discussions of various versions of the subgenre, see also Lennard J. Davis, *Resisting Novels: Ideology and Fiction* (New York: Methuen, 1987), Chapter 7 (what Howe calls the "political novel," Davis refers to as the "novel of political content"); and Paula Rabinowitz, *Labor and Desire: Women's Revolutionary Fiction in Depression America* (Chapel Hill: University of North Carolina Press, 1991), pp. 73-78.

6. On the division in certain types of literature between the private and the public, and between the individual and the collective, see Barbara Foley, *Radical Representations: Politics and Form in U.S. Proletarian Fiction, 1929-1941* (Durham, NC: Duke University Press, 1993), pp. 346-348; and Davis, *Resisting Novels,* pp. 231-232. Although Davis and Foley are discussing the novel in these studies, their analyses strike me as being applicable to drama as well. As Davis points out, collectivity can be represented on the stage much more readily than in the pages of a novel; as I will be arguing, however, and as Davis's discussion of the novel suggests,

the technological ability of drama to represent collectivity tends to collapse in the face of the privatizing imperatives of the love story. For an excellent discussion of the love story in the novel, one which has also informed my thinking here, see Joseph Allen Boone, *Tradition Counter Tradition: Love and the Form of Fiction* (Chicago, IL: University of Chicago Press, 1987).

7. D.A. Miller, *Narrative and Its Discontents: Problems of Closure in the Traditional Novel* (Princeton, NJ: Princeton University Press, 1981), p. 5. Miller distinguishes "closure" from "ending": closure, he argues, "refers us better, I think, to the *functions* of an ending: to justify the cessation of narrative and to complete the meaning of what has gone before" (p. xi, footnote 2).

8. For a useful summary of theories of the "open-ended" narrative see Boone, *Tradition Counter Tradition,* p. 146. Although the kind of text I imagine here differs from the indeterminacy of the classic open-ended narrative through its decisive promotion of political struggle, it resembles these narratives to the extent´ that the reader is, as Boone summarizes, "forced to engage with the text beyond its actual close" (p. 146). On closure and the "politics plot," see also Foley, *Radical Representations,* pp. 346-348.

9. For a related discussion of the conflict between "the personal" and "the political" in AIDS film, see Bart Beaty, "The Syndrome is the System: A Political Reading of *Longtime Companion,*" in *Fluid Exchanges: Artists and Critics in the AIDS Crisis,* ed. James Miller (Toronto: University of Toronto Press, 1992), pp. 111-121.

10. See, for instance, John Clum, *Acting Gay: Male Homosexuality in Modern Drama,* Revised Edition (New York: Columbia University Press, 1994), especially pp. 76 and 313.

11. A plot summary of *The Normal Heart* is provided in Chapter 2 of this book.

12. Analyses that take a supportive stance toward Kramer's play include Randy Shilts, *And the Band Played On: Politics, People, and the AIDS Epidemic* (New York, Penguin, 1988), pp. 556-557; D.S. Lawson, "Rage and Remembrance: The AIDS Plays," in *AIDS: The Literary Response,* ed. Emmanuel S. Nelson (New York: Twayne Publishers, 1992), pp. 141-143; and Joseph Papp's foreword to the published version of the play. The play also received a number of positive reviews in the mainstream press.

13. See, for instance, Douglas Crimp, "How to Have Promiscuity in an Epidemic," in *AIDS: Cultural Analysis/Cultural Activism,* ed. Douglas Crimp (Cambridge, MA: MIT Press, 1988), pp. 246-252; David Román, "Performing All Our Lives: AIDS, Performance, Community," in *Critical Theory and Performance,* eds. Janelle G. Reinelt and Joseph R. Roach (Ann Arbor: University of Michigan Press, 1992), pp. 208-211; Mark Caldwell, "The Literature of AIDS: Sensationalism, Hysteria, and Good Sense," *Dissent* 37 (1990):344; Richard Goldstein, "Kramer's Complaint," *Village Voice,* July 2, 1985:20, 22; Brandon Judell, "Scenery Chewing and Other Choice Words," *Advocate,* May 28, 1985:41-42; and David Bergman, *Gaiety Transfigured: Gay Self-Representation in American Literature* (Madison: University of Wisconsin Press, 1991), Chapter 7. Kramer has responded to a number

of these criticisms in *Reports*, pp. 91-94. On Kramer's rocky history with GMHC, see again Chapter 2.

14. Crimp's and Román's pieces are especially compelling and specifically address my central concern with the political effects of the use of dominant forms. See especially Crimp, "How to Have Promiscuity," p. 248; and Román, "Performing All Our Lives," pp. 209-210.

15. See Crimp and the individuals quoted in Judell. Reviewers got bogged down in this question of "authenticity" as well, criticizing *The Normal Heart* for mixing "fact and fiction" (Barnes) or for making complaints about the early years of the epidemic that were no longer justified in 1985. See Clive Barnes, review of *The Normal Heart* by Larry Kramer, *New York Post*, May 4, 1985; reprinted in *New York Theatre Critics' Reviews* 1985:280; Gerald Weales, review of *The Normal Heart* by Larry Kramer, *Commonweal*, July 12, 1985:407. *New York Theatre Critics' Reviews* volumes will be herein referred to as NYTCR.

16. Bergman, *Gaiety Transfigured*, pp. 134-135. After criticizing *The Normal Heart*'s endorsement of marriage and family, Bergman argues that Kramer "only belatedly realizes [in *Reports from the Holocaust*] that the worst enemies of the homosexual are those, like Adolf Eichmann, who act to protect the family." Bergman, *Gaiety Transfigured*, p. 135.

17. Larry Kramer, *The Normal Heart* (New York: Plume, 1985), p. 38. All further references will appear in the body of the text.

18. Kramer, "1,112 and Counting," *Reports*, pp. 33-51. The article was reprinted in gay papers around the country.

19. "I tried to make Ned Weeks as obnoxious as I could," Kramer has written. "He isn't my idea of a hero. He fucks up totally. He yells at his dying lover and screams and rants and raves at and against everyone and everything else and gets tossed out of 'the organization' on his ass. I was trying, somehow and again, to atone for my own behavior." *Reports*, p. 93. Such a position is supported by the fact that other characters in the play are quick to denounce Ned for his hypocrisy in advocating celibacy while taking a lover.

20. On Kramer's reliance on audience empathy, see again Román, "Performing All Our Lives," p. 209.

21. Papp, foreword to *The Normal Heart*, p. 29.

22. William A. Henry III, review of *The Normal Heart* by Larry Kramer, *Time*, May 13, 1985; reprinted in NYTCR 1985:281.

23. One of the three scenes following Ned's removal from the board consists of a conversation between Felix and Ben, but the two men discuss Felix and Ned's relationship extensively.

24. Román, "Performing All Our Lives," p. 209. See also Seymour Kleinberg, "Life After Death," *The New Republic*, August 11 and 18, 1986:30.

25. Clum, *Acting Gay*, p. 76.

26. Román, "Performing All Our Lives," p. 210.

27. These instances include Scene 5, in which the volunteers of the nascent organization meet in Ned's apartment and elect Bruce their president; Scene 9, in which members of the board of the organization meet with a representative of the

mayor's office at City Hall; and Scene 11, which depicts board members and volunteers struggling to accommodate a growing need for services despite understaffing and an overcrowded office. Scene 5 turns into a romantic comedy of errors, as various characters make passes at one another; Ned entirely dominates Scene 9; and Scene 11 is organized around two bravura speeches by members of the AIDS organization, both of which focus on sex and love. Crimp has gone so far as to argue, in fact, that "*The Normal Heart* is a purely personal—*not* a political—drama, a drama of a few heroic individuals in the AIDS movement" (Crimp, "How to Have Promiscuity," p. 248).

28. Crimp, "How to Have Promiscuity," p. 248.

29. William A. Henry III, review of *Millennium Approaches* by Tony Kushner, *Time*, May 17, 1993; reprinted in NYTCR 1993:212. See also David Richards, "Visions of Heaven and Hell," *The New York Times*, May 16, 1993: sec. 2, pp. H1, H7.

30. Michael Feingold, review of *Perestroika* by Tony Kushner, *Village Voice*, December 7, 1993; reprinted in NYTCR 1993:394.

31. David Savran, "Ambivalence, Utopia, and a Queer Sort of Materialism: How *Angels in America* Reconstructs the Nation," *Theatre Journal* 47 (1995):222.

32. Kushner, *Millennium Approaches*, pp. 89-90.

33. Kushner, *Perestroika*, p.36. All further references will appear in the body of the text.

34. On liberalism and identity politics in *Angels in America*, see Savran, "Ambivalence,"especially pp. 219-224.

35. Gordon Rogoff, "Angels in America, Devils in the Wings," *Theater* 24, no. 2 (1993):29.

36. Walter Olson, review of *Perestroika* by Tony Kushner, *National Review*, January 24, 1994:72. See also Feingold, review of *Perestroika*, NYTCR 1993: 394; and David Richards, review of *Perestroika* by Tony Kushner, *The New York Times*, November 28, 1993: sec. 2, p. 27.

37. Kushner, *Millennium Approaches*, p. 14.

38. As the characters in the epilogue explain, a fountain sprung up in Jerusalem where the angel Bethesda touched her foot, and "if anyone who was suffering, in the body or the spirit, walked through the waters of the fountain of Bethesda, they would be healed, washed clean of pain" (p. 147).

39. Robert Brustein, review of *Perestroika* by Tony Kushner, *New Republic*, December 27, 1993; reprinted in NYTCR 1993:392; Linda Winer, review of *Perestroika* by Tony Kushner, *New York Newsday*, November 24, 1993; reprinted in NYTCR 1993:391. For a scholarly analysis that takes a similar approach, see Charles McNulty, "*Angels in America*: Tony Kushner's Theses on the Philosophy of History," *Modern Drama* 39 (1996):93.

40. Kushner, introduction to *Perestroika*, p. 8; Frank Rich, review of *Perestroika* by Tony Kushner, *The New York Times*, November 24, 1993:C11.

41. I include "the bourgeois family" here, for although alienated from her son and her daughter-in-law during the course of the play, Hannah is shown to

have discovered a new family of choice (to borrow Kath Weston's phrase) after she assists Prior when he becomes sick in the Mormon visitors' center.

42. Linda Winer, review of *Millennium Approaches* by Tony Kushner, *New York Newsday*, May 5, 1993; reprinted in NYTCR 1993:209.

43. Schulman's last lines in *People in Trouble* perform a function uncannily similar to Prior's final speech in Kushner's play. As we have just seen, Prior's comment that the "Great Work Begins" serves to focus attention back on the audience, reminding them that the "Great Work" to which the angel referred is not the tasks Prior himself performs—or even Kushner's play itself—but the work that will occur outside the theater doors. Schulman offers her readers a similarly open ending—one that becomes possible only once Kate leaves Peter and Molly leaves Kate. *People in Trouble* concludes with Molly, James, and other members of Justice gathering at James's apartment before going to a demonstration at St. Vincent's Hospital. James complains that "We are a people in trouble. We do not act," at which point Schulman concludes her novel with the words, "Then everyone went to Saint Vincent's because there was nothing more to say." Justice ends its meeting, and Schulman her novel, with these words, because both parties realize that discussing a subject can only do so much good. Neither talking nor writing novels is enough, Schulman insists: now that there is "nothing more to say," both her characters and her readers must go out and act. Sarah Schulman, *People in Trouble* (New York: Dutton, 1990), p. 228.

44. I am indebted here to D.A. Miller's understanding of what he calls the "traditional novel," especially as concerns the question of narrative closure. See Miller, *Narrative and Its Discontents*, especially p. 109.

45. For an excellent discussion of the public health implications of the breakdown of this collapse between the public and the private, see Ronald Bayer, *Private Acts, Social Consequences: AIDS and the Politics of Public Health* (New York: The Free Press, 1989).

46. Schulman's use of what she termed a "social realist" style for her novel renders love and politics as incompatible in *People in Trouble* as they are in the writings of the men. Interestingly enough, however, Schulman's adoption of a realist style was unusual for her fictional writings and had to do with her desire to convey her polemic clearly to her audience. "I've published five novels," she explained, "and that's the only one that's written in that form because I was trying to explain a political idea, so I used this very flat surface texture and this very conventional structure . . . to try to get this idea across." (Sarah Schulman, telephone interview). Moreover, when it comes time to decide between love or political struggle, *People in Trouble* demonstrates little of the ambivalence that Kramer's and Kushner's texts do.

Chapter 4

1. Darrell Yates Rist, "The Deadly Cost of an Obsession," *The Nation*, February 13, 1989; quotes are from pp. 196 and 200 respectively.

2. Darrell Yates Rist, "Reply," *The Nation*, March 20, 1989:392.

3. Robin Hardy, "Die Harder," *Village Voice*, July 2, 1991:33.

4. Frank Browning, "Turf Wars," *Village Voice,* July 10, 1990:18.

5. Here, of course, I am defining politics more broadly than in my other chapters, to include cultural politics as well as contests with the state. See my initial definition in the "Goals" section of Chapter 1.

6. Claims for the uniqueness of gay men and lesbians coming together to do political work concerning AIDS obviously ignore the extent to which such a process has occurred throughout the epidemic on political as well as service levels, as Cindy Patton and others have noted. At the same time, however, such comments accurately describe the experiences of a number ACT UP women with extensive backgrounds in political organizing, who observed that ACT UP represented one of the first times that they had worked with gay men on grassroots activism. See Cindy Patton, *Inventing AIDS* (New York: Routledge, 1990), Chapter 1.

7. This is not to say that finding a sense of community was not important to ACT UP/New York members, who frequently socialized with one another in small groups. Rather, what I am trying to do here is to account for why Rhode Island activists tended to emphasize community formation and de-emphasize dating when discussing why the group was important to them, in contrast to their New York counterparts, who stressed the importance of both.

8. Social support networks have always been important within progressive organizing. For a classic study of this phenomenon, see Blanche Wiesen Cook, "Female Support Networks and Political Activism: Lillian Wald, Crystal Eastman, Emma Goldman," *Chrysalis,* No. 3 (1977):43-61.

Appendix

1. Michael Frisch, "Oral History and *Hard Times:* A Review Essay," in *A Shared Authority: Essays on the Craft and Meaning of Oral and Public History* (Albany: State University of New York Press, 1990), p. 10.

2. In this respect, I am not alone among scholars of lesbian and gay history. Elizabeth Lapovsky Kennedy, for instance, has called for a balancing of skepticism about the usefulness of "the evidence of experience" in establishing historical fact with a realization that without the accumulation of and reliance on this kind of evidence, we will end up knowing very little about the truth of lesbian and gay lives. Elizabeth Lapovsky Kennedy, "Telling Tales: Oral History and the Construction of Pre-Stonewall Lesbian History," *Radical History Review* No. 62 (Spring 1995):76, n. 4. "The Evidence of Experience" is the title of an extremely influential article on this topic by Joan Scott. See Joan Scott, "The Evidence of Experience," in *The Lesbian and Gay Studies Reader,* eds. Henry Abelove, Michèle Aina Barale, and David M. Halperin (New York: Routledge, 1993), pp. 397-415.

3. Micaela di Leonardo, "Oral History as Ethnographic Encounter," *Oral History Review* 15 (Spring 1987):3.

4. At the time I did my research, both archives were in the possession of their respective ACT UP chapters.

5. Internal memos produced for consumption at meetings and discussion about ACT UP in gay publications did address these conflicts and crises directly, and I draw on these kinds of documents throughout my discussion.

6. Jane Sherron De Hart, "Oral Sources and Contemporary History: Dispelling Old Assumptions," *Journal of American History* 80 (September 1993):591; Kennedy, "Telling Tales," pp. 63-65. See also David King Dunaway, "Field Recording Oral History," *Oral History Review* 15 (Spring 1987):37. As Kennedy notes of the interviews of older lesbians she conducted with Madeline D. Davis, "As we listened to and worked with these oral narratives, we realized that these stories were not told for the first time to us, the oral historians, but that they had been shared before with friends at parties and in bars. . . . This made sense to us because working-class lesbians spent a lot of time socializing together in explicitly lesbian space. Their lives were defined by finding and supporting other lesbians in a hostile environment and by developing strategies to live with some dignity and pride. What better way to accomplish this than by sharing stories about these successes and defeats." Kennedy, "Telling Tales," pp. 63-64.

7. As Frisch has noted, all oral history narrators provide to a certain extent their own narrative, theoretical, and historical frameworks for understanding their experiences. Interpretation is rarely left entirely to the interviewer. See Michael Frisch, "Oral History and the Presentation of Class Consciousness: The *New York Times* v. The Buffalo Unemployed," in *A Shared Authority,* pp. 63-64.

8. My use of the term "narrators" to describe the people I interviewed is borrowed from Elizabeth Lapovsky Kennedy and Madeline D. Davis, *Boots of Leather, Slippers of Gold: The History of a Lesbian Community* (New York: Penguin, 1994).

9. Judith Stacey defines "the ethnographic method" as "intensive participant-observation study that yields a synthetic cultural account." Judith Stacey, "Can There Be a Feminist Ethnography?" in *Women's Words: The Feminist Practice of Oral History,* eds. Sherna Berger Gluck and Daphne Patai (New York: Routledge, 1991), p. 112.

10. di Leonardo, "Oral History," pp. 4-5. It is important to note that, to the extent that my involvement with ACT UP/RI preceded my decision to study the group by a number of years, my work with ACT UP/RI can only be considered "participant observation" in the loosest sense. ACT UP/RI was my object of study, but it was also an important part of my own life. For one historian's discussion of the advantages of and problems inherent in researching a movement with which one has been personally involved, see Sara Evans, *Personal Politics: The Roots of Women's Liberation in the Civil Rights Movement and the New Left* (New York: Vintage, 1980), pp. x-xi. As Evans ultimately concludes, "The rapport that developed in many interviews resulted in part from my own and my informants' confidence that my prior research and my personal experience together allowed me to comprehend what they had to say in a way that no 'outsider' could. The results, time after time, were extraordinary."

11. Dunaway, "Field Recording Oral History," pp. 28-29; di Leonardo, "Oral History," p. 13.

12. di Leonardo, "Oral History," p. 6.

13. Esther Newton's book *Cherry Grove* provides a model in this regard. Although Newton relies on the memories of others for most of her history of the Grove, she also found it invaluable that she was there herself for a small piece of the history she recounts. See Esther Newton, *Cherry Grove, Fire Island: Sixty Years in America's First Gay and Lesbian Town* (Boston: Beacon Press, 1993), especially p. 303.

14. See, for instance, Michael Frisch, "Preparing Interview Transcripts for Documentary Publication: A Line-by-Line Illustration of the Editing Process," in *A Shared Authority*, pp. 84-86.

Bibliography

Abelove, Henry, Michèle Aina Barale, and David M. Halperin, eds. *The Lesbian and Gay Studies Reader.* New York: Routledge, 1993.

ACT UP/Network. *Universal Health Care: A Handbook for Activists.* Los Angeles, CA: ACT UP/Network, 1991.

"ACT UP/New York Capsule History." ACT UP New York Web site, www.actupny.org.

Agnew, Jean-Christophe. "The Consuming Vision of Henry James." In eds. Richard Wightman Fox and T. J. Jackson Lears, *The Culture of Consumption: Critical Essays in American History, 1880-1980* (New York: Pantheon Books, 1983), pp. 65-100.

"AIDS Movement and Its Challenge, The." *Radical America* 21 (November/December 1988):61-63.

Arn, Tony and Gunther Freehill. "Demanding Universal Health Care." In ACT UP/Network, *Universal Health Care: A Handbook for Activists* (Los Angeles, CA: ACT UP Network, 1991), pp. 3-4.

Barnes, Clive. Review of *The Normal Heart,* by Larry Kramer. *New York Post,* May 4, 1985. Reprinted in *New York Theatre Critics' Reviews* 1985:280.

"Battle Fatigue." *New Yorker,* November 9, 1992:39-40.

Baudrillard, Jean. "Consumer Society." In ed. Mark Poster, *Selected Writings* (Stanford, CA: Stanford University Press, 1988), pp. 29-56.

Bawer, Bruce. *A Place at the Table: The Gay Individual in American Society.* New York: Poseidon, 1993.

Bayer, Ronald. *Private Acts, Social Consequences: AIDS and the Politics of Public Health.* New York: The Free Press, 1989.

Beaty, Bart. "The Syndrome is the System: A Political Reading of *Longtime Companion.*" In ed. James Miller, *Fluid Exchanges: Artists and Critics in the AIDS Crisis* (Toronto: University of Toronto Press, 1992), pp. 111-121.

Bell, Stephanie. "'Galpals' and 'Space Alien Drag Queens': Outing, AIDS and Tabloid Newspapers." *Radical America* 25 (January-March 1991):73-96.

Bergman, David. *Gaiety Transfigured: Gay Self-Representation in American Literature.* Madison: University of Wisconsin Press, 1991.

Biddle, Frederic M. "ACT UP's Last Act?" *Boston Globe Magazine,* September 5, 1993:13, 25-28.

Boone, Joseph Allen. *Tradition Counter Tradition: Love and the Form of Fiction.* Chicago, IL: University of Chicago Press, 1987.

Brown, Wendy. "Finding the Man in the State." *Feminist Studies* 18 (Spring 1992): 7-34.

Browning, Frank. "Turf Wars." *Village Voice,* July 10, 1990:17-18.

Brustein, Robert. Review of *Perestroika,* by Tony Kushner. *New Republic,* December 27, 1993. Reprinted in *New York Theatre Critics' Reviews* 1993:392-393.

Burkett, Elinor. *The Gravest Show on Earth: America in the Age of AIDS.* Boston, MA: Houghton Mifflin, 1995.

Caldwell, Mark. "The Literature of AIDS: Sensationalism, Hysteria, and Good Sense." *Dissent* 37 (1990):342-347.

Campbell, Courtney S. "Ethics and Militant AIDS Activism." In ed. Frederic G. Reamer, *AIDS and Ethics* (New York: Columbia University Press, 1991), pp. 155-187.

Carroll, Jon. "One White Guy Sittin' Around Rantin'." *San Francisco Chronicle,* July 3, 1991:E10.

Carter, George M. *ACT UP, the AIDS War and Activism.* Open Magazine Pamphlet Series no. 15 (Westfield, NJ: Open Magazine, 1992).

Chew, Sally. "What's Going Down with ACT UP?" *Out,* November 1993:72-75, 130-137.

"Civil Disobedience vs. Uncivilized Behavior." Editorial. *New York Daily News,* December 12, 1989:28.

Clum, John. "'And Once I Had It All': AIDS Narratives and Memories of an American Dream." In eds. Timothy F. Murphy and Suzanne Poirier, *Writing AIDS: Gay Literature, Language, and Analysis* (New York: Columbia University Press, 1993), pp. 200-224.

————. *Acting Gay: Male Homosexuality in Modern Drama.* Revised Edition. New York: Columbia University Press, 1994.

Cohen, Carl. "Militant Morality: Civil Disobedience and Bioethics." *Hastings Center Report,* November/December 1989:23-25.

Cohen, Cathy Jean. "Power, Resistance and the Construction of Crisis: Marginalized Communities Respond to AIDS." PhD dissertation, University of Michigan, 1993.

Cook, Blanche Wiesen. "Female Support Networks and Political Activism: Lillian Wald, Crystal Eastman, Emma Goldman." *Chrysalis* 3 (1977):43-61.

Corea, Gena. *The Invisible Epidemic: The Story of Women and AIDS.* New York: HarperCollins, 1992.

Craig, Scott. Letter. *OutWeek,* January 14, 1990:7.

Crenshaw, Kimberlé Williams. "Race, Reform, and Retrenchment: Transformation and Legitimation in Antidiscrimination Law." *Harvard Law Review* 101 (May 1988):1331-1387.

Crimp, Douglas, ed. *AIDS: Cultural Analysis/Cultural Activism.* Cambridge, MA: MIT Press, 1988.

————. "How to Have Promiscuity in an Epidemic." In ed. Douglas Crimp, *AIDS: Cultural Analysis/Cultural Activism* (Cambridge, MA: MIT Press, 1988), pp. 237-271.

Crimp, Douglas with Adam Rolston. *AIDS Demo Graphics.* Seattle, WA: Bay Press, 1990.

Daniels, Norman. *Seeking Fair Treatment: From the AIDS Epidemic to National Health Care Reform.* New York: Oxford University Press, 1995.

Davis, Lennard J. *Resisting Novels: Ideology and Fiction.* New York: Methuen, 1987.

De Hart, Jane Sherron. "Oral Sources and Contemporary History: Dispelling Old Assumptions." *Journal of American History* 80 (1993):582-595.

di Leonardo, Micaela. "Oral History as Ethnographic Encounter." *Oral History Review* 15 (Spring 1987):1-20.

"Duberman Addresses Stonewall Dedication." *OutWeek,* June 26, 1989:20-21.

Duggan, Lisa. "The Discipline Problem: Queer Theory Meets Lesbian and Gay History." *GLQ* 2 (1995):179-191.

Dunaway, David King. "Field Recording Oral History." *Oral History Review* 15 (Spring 1987):21-42.

Elbaz, Gilbert. "The Sociology of AIDS Activism: The Case of ACT UP/New York, 1987-1992." PhD dissertation, City University of New York, 1992.

Epstein, Barbara. *Political Protest and Cultural Revolution: Nonviolent Direct Action in the 1970s and 1980s.* Berkeley: University of California Press, 1991.

Epstein, Steven. *Impure Science: AIDS, Activism, and the Politics of Knowledge.* Berkeley: University of California Press, 1996.

Erni, John Nguyet. *Unstable Frontiers: Technomedicine and the Cultural Politics of "Curing" AIDS.* Minneapolis: University of Minnesota Press, 1994.

Ervolino, Bill. "ACT UP Making Headlines—and Enemies." *The (Hackensack) Record,* February 10, 1993:A6.

Evans, Sara. *Personal Politics: The Roots of Women's Liberation in the Civil Rights Movement and the New Left.* New York: Vintage, 1980.

Fee, Elizabeth and Daniel M. Fox, eds. *AIDS: The Making of a Chronic Disease.* Berkeley: University of California Press, 1992.

Feingold, Michael. Review of *Perestroika,* by Tony Kushner. *Village Voice,* December 7, 1993. Reprinted in *New York Theatre Critics' Reviews* 1993:393-394.

Field, Nicola. *Over the Rainbow: Money, Class, and Homophobia.* London: Pluto Press, 1995.

Foley, Barbara. *Radical Representations: Politics and Form in U.S. Proletarian Fiction, 1929-1941.* Durham, NC: Duke University Press, 1993.

Ford, Dave. "A.I.D.S.: Words from the Front." *Spin,* January 1989:60-62, 76.

Fox, Richard Wightman and T. J. Jackson Lears, eds. *The Culture of Consumption: Critical Essays in American History, 1880-1980.* New York: Pantheon Books, 1983.

Freitas, Anthony, Susan Kaiser, and Tania Hammidi. "Communities, Commodities, Cultural Space, and Style." In ed. Daniel L. Wardlow, *Gays, Lesbians, and Consumer Behavior: Theory, Practice, and Research Issues in Marketing* (Binghamton, NY: Harrington Park Press, 1996), pp. 83-107.

Freyer, Felice J. "ACT-UP Rallies Against AIDS Tracking Policy." *Providence Journal Bulletin,* October 21, 1993:D17.

Frisch, Michael. *A Shared Authority: Essays on the Craft and Meaning of Oral and Public History.* Albany: State University of New York Press, 1990.

Fuss, Diana, ed. *Inside/Out: Lesbian Theories, Gay Theories.* New York: Routledge, 1991.

————."Inside/Out." In ed. Diana Fuss, *Inside/Out: Lesbian Theories, Gay Theories* (New York: Routledge, 1991), pp. 1-10.

Gamson, Joshua. "Silence, Death, and the Invisible Enemy: AIDS Activism and Social Movement 'Newness.'" In Michael Burawoy et. al., *Ethnography Unbound: Power and Resistance in the Modern Metropolis* (Berkeley: University of California Press, 1991), pp. 35-57.

Gluck, Sherna Berger and Daphne Patai, eds. *Women's Words: The Feminist Practice of Oral History.* New York: Routledge, 1991.

Gluckman, Amy and Betsy Reed, eds. *Homo Economics: Capitalism, Community, and Lesbian and Gay Life.* New York: Routledge, 1997.

Golden, Mark. "ACT UP Redux." *QW*, October 11, 1992:22-25.

Goldstein, Richard. "Kramer's Complaint." *Village Voice*, July 2, 1985:20, 22.

Grover, Jan Zita. "AIDS: Keywords." In ed. Douglas Crimp, *AIDS: Cultural Analysis/Cultural Activism* (Cambridge, MA: MIT Press, 1988), pp. 17-30.

"Haitians with HIV Are Being Murdered in a U.S. Military Concentration Camp." ACT UP/New York document, 1993, ACT UP/New York archives.

Hardy, Robin. "Die Harder." *Village Voice*, July 2, 1991:33-34.

Harrington, Mark. "A Fifth Anniversary Letter to ACT UP." March 9, 1992, ACT UP/New York archives.

_____. "Let My People In." *OutWeek*, August 8, 1990:34-35, 37.

Harvey, David. *The Condition of Postmodernity: An Enquiry into the Origins of Cultural Change.* Cambridge, MA: Blackwell, 1990.

Henry, William A., III. Review of *The Normal Heart*, by Larry Kramer. *Time*, May 13, 1985. Reprinted in *New York Theatre Critics' Reviews* 1985:281.

_____. Review of *Millennium Approaches*, by Tony Kushner. *Time*, May 17, 1993. Reprinted in *New York Theatre Critics' Reviews* 1993:212.

Howe, Irving. *Politics and the Novel.* 1957. New York: Columbia University Press, 1992.

Hummel, Jim. "AIDS Activists Protest Bill of Rights Display." *Providence Journal*, October 21, 1990:B1, B11.

Hunter, Nan D. "Marriage, Law, and Gender: A Feminist Inquiry." *Law and Sexuality: A Review of Lesbian and Gay Legal Issues* 1 (Summer 1991):9-30.

Jay, Karla and Allen Young, eds. *Out of the Closets: Voices of Gay Liberation.* Twentieth Anniversary Edition. New York: New York University Press, 1992.

Jones, Therese, ed. *Sharing the Delirium: Second Generation AIDS Plays and Performances.* Portsmouth, NH: Heinemann, 1994.

Judell, Brandon. "Scenery Chewing and Other Choice Words." *Advocate*, May 28, 1985:41-42.

Kayal, Philip M. *Bearing Witness: Gay Men's Health Crisis and the Politics of AIDS.* Boulder, CO: Westview Press, 1993.

Kennedy, Elizabeth Lapovsky. "Telling Tales: Oral History and the Construction of Pre-Stonewall Lesbian History." *Radical History Review* No. 62 (Spring 1995):59-79.

Kennedy, Elizabeth Lapovsky and Madeline D. Davis. *Boots of Leather, Slippers of Gold: The History of a Lesbian Community.* New York: Penguin, 1994.

Kerrison, Ray. Column. *New York Post*, December 15, 1989:2.

King, Martin Luther, Jr. "Letter from Birmingham City Jail." Philadelphia: American Friends Service Committee, May 1963.

Kleinberg, Seymour. "Life After Death." *The New Republic*, August 11 and 18, 1986:28-33.

Kolata, Gina. "Advocates' Tactics on AIDS Issues Provoking Warnings of a Backlash." *New York Times,* March 11, 1990: sec. 4, p. 5.

Kramer, Larry. *The Normal Heart.* New York: Plume, 1985.

————. *Reports from the Holocaust: The Story of an AIDS Activist.* Updated and Expanded Edition. New York: St. Martin's Press, 1994.

Kruger, Steven F. *AIDS Narratives: Gender and Sexuality, Fiction and Science.* New York: Garland, 1996.

Kushner, Tony. *Angels in America: Millennium Approaches.* New York: Theatre Communications Group, 1993.

————. *Angels in America: Perestroika.* New York: Theatre Communications Group, 1994.

"Larry Kramer." *Current Biography,* March 1994:20-24.

Lawson, D.S. "Rage and Remembrance: The AIDS Plays." In ed. Emmanuel S. Nelson, *AIDS: The Literary Response* (New York: Twayne Publishers, 1992), pp. 140-154.

Leo, John. "When Activism Becomes Gangsterism." *U.S. News and World Report,* February 5, 1990:18.

Loewenstein, Andrea Freud. "Troubled Times" (interview with Sarah Schulman). *Women's Review of Books,* July 1990:22-23.

Maggenti, Maria. "No Half Measures" (interview with Paul Monette). *OutWeek,* May 8, 1991:56-58.

Marx, Karl. *Capital: A Critique of Political Economy.* Volume 1. 1887. New York: International Publishers, 1967.

McClintock Project Working Group (ACT UP/New York). *The Barbara McClintock Project to Cure AIDS,* 1993.

McNulty, Charles. "*Angels in America*: Tony Kushner's Theses on the Philosophy of History." *Modern Drama* 39 (1996):84-96.

McPhillips, Jody. "ACT UP! Protests at Journal." *Providence Journal Bulletin,* December 16, 1993:D19.

Meluci, Alberto. *Nomads of the Present: Social Movements and Individual Needs in Contemporary Society.* Eds. John Keane and Paul Mier. (Philadelphia, PA: Temple University Press, 1989).

————. "The Symbolic Challenge of Contemporary Movements." *Social Research* 52 (1985):789-816.

Meluci, Alberto, John Keane, and Paul Mier. "New Perspectives on Social Movements: An Interview with Alberto Melucci." In Melucci, eds. John Keane and Paul Mier, *Nomads of the Present: Social Movements and Individual Needs in Contemporary Society* (Philadelphia, PA: Temple University Press, 1989), pp. 180-232.

Meredith, Linda. Letter. *OutWeek,* August 22, 1990:5.

Meyer, Richard. "Rock Hudson's Body." In ed. Diana Fuss, *Inside/Out: Lesbian Theories, Gay Theories* (New York: Routledge, 1991), pp. 259-288.

Miller, Andrew and Rex Wockner. "AIDS/Abortion Rights Demo Halts High Mass at St. Pat's." *OutWeek,* December 24, 1989:12-18, 20.

Miller, D.A. *Narrative and Its Discontents: Problems of Closure in the Traditional Novel.* Princeton, NJ: Princeton University Press, 1981.

Miller, James, ed. *Fluid Exchanges: Artists and Critics in the AIDS Crisis.* Toronto: University of Toronto Press, 1992.

Mohr, Richard D. *Gay Ideas: Outing and Other Controversies.* Boston, MA: Beacon Press, 1992.

Monette, Paul. *Afterlife.* New York: Crown Publishers, Inc., 1990.

————. *Becoming a Man: Half a Life Story.* New York: Harcourt Brace Jovanovich, 1992.

————. *Borrowed Time: An AIDS Memoir.* New York: Harcourt Brace Jovanovich, 1988.

————. *Last Watch of the Night: Essays Too Personal and Otherwise.* New York: Harcourt Brace and Company, 1994.

Morgan, Tracy D. Letter. *OutWeek,* August 22, 1990:6.

Murphy, Timothy F. and Suzanne Poirier, eds. *Writing AIDS: Gay Literature, Language, and Analysis.* New York: Columbia University Press, 1993.

Nelson, Emmanuel S., ed. *AIDS: The Literary Response.* New York: Twayne Publishers, 1992.

————, ed. *Contemporary Gay American Novelists: A Bio-Bibliographical Critical Sourcebook.* Westport, CT: Greenwood Press, 1993.

Newton, Esther. *Cherry Grove, Fire Island: Sixty Years in America's First Gay and Lesbian Town.* Boston: Beacon Press, 1993.

Novick, Alvin. "Civil Disobedience in Time of AIDS," *Hastings Center Reports,* November/December 1989:35-36.

Nussbaum, Bruce. *Good Intentions: How Big Business and the Medical Establishment Are Corrupting the Fight Against AIDS, Alzheimer's, Cancer, and More.* New York: Penguin, 1991.

Olson, Walter. Review of *Perestroika,* by Tony Kushner. *National Review,* January 24, 1994:71-73.

O'Neil, Cliff. "Demonstrators Rain Fire and Brimstone on NIH Headquarters." *OutWeek,* June 6, 1990:14-16.

"Over Whose Dead Bodies?" Editorial. *OutWeek,* December 24, 1989:4.

Padgug, Robert A. and Gerald M. Oppenheimer. "Riding the Tiger: AIDS and the Gay Community." In eds. Elizabeth Fee and Daniel M. Fox, *AIDS: The Making of a Chronic Disease* (Berkeley: University of California Press, 1992), pp. 245-278.

Patton, Cindy. *Inventing AIDS.* New York: Routledge, 1990.

————. *Last Served?: Gendering the HIV Pandemic.* London: Taylor and Francis, 1994.

Pepper, Rachel. "Schism Slices ACT UP in Two." *OutWeek,* October 10, 1990:12-14.

Piven, Frances Fox and Richard A. Cloward. *Poor People's Movements: Why They Succeed, How They Fail.* New York: Vintage, 1979.

POZ, March 1997 (special issue on ACT UP).

Presidential Debate Transcript. *The New York Times,* October 12, 1992:14-17.

Prevost, Lisa. "ACT UP Leery of Reduction in Anonymous HIV Testing Sites." *Newpaper* (Providence), April 4, 1991:2.

Rabinowitz, Paula. *Labor and Desire: Women's Revolutionary Fiction in Depression America.* Chapel Hill: University of North Carolina Press, 1991.

Reamer, Frederic G., ed. *AIDS and Ethics.* New York: Columbia University Press, 1991.

Reinelt, Janelle G. and Joseph R. Roach, eds. *Critical Theory and Performance.* Ann Arbor: University of Michigan Press, 1992.

Reyes, Nina. "ACT UP T and D Plans Spinoff." *NYQ,* November 24, 1991:9.

————. "Hundreds of Women Storm CDC over AIDS Definition." *OutWeek,* December 19, 1990:16-17.

Rich, Frank. Review of *Perestroika,* by Tony Kushner. *The New York Times,* November 24, 1993:C11, C20.

Richards, David. Review of *Perestroika,* by Tony Kushner. *The New York Times,* November 28, 1993: sec. 2, pp. 1, 27.

————. "Visions of Heaven and Hell." *The New York Times,* May 16, 1993: sec. 2, pp. H1, H7.

Rist, Darrell Yates. "Reply." *The Nation,* March 20, 1989:382, 392.

————. "The Deadly Costs of an Obsession." *The Nation,* February 13, 1989: 181, 196-200.

Rofes, Eric. *Reviving the Tribe: Regenerating Gay Men's Sexuality and Culture in the Ongoing Epidemic.* Binghamton, NY: Harrington Park Press, 1996.

Rogoff, Gordon. "Angels in America, Devils in the Wings." *Theater* 24, no. 2 (1993):21-29.

Román, David. "Paul Monette." In ed. Emmanuel S. Nelson, *Contemporary Gay American Novelists: A Bio-Bibliographical Critical Sourcebook* (Westport, CT: Greenwood Press, 1993), pp. 272-281.

————. "Performing All Our Lives: AIDS, Performance, Community." In eds. Janelle G. Reinelt and Joseph R. Roach, *Critical Theory and Performance* (Ann Arbor: University of Michigan Press, 1992), pp. 208-221.

Rubin, Gayle with Judith Butler. "Sexual Traffic." *differences* 6 (Summer-Fall 1994):62-99.

Savran, David. "Ambivalence, Utopia, and a Queer Sort of Materialism: How *Angels in America* Reconstructs the Nation." *Theatre Journal* 47 (1995):207-227.

Scott, Joan. "The Evidence of Experience." In eds. Henry Abelove, Michèle Aina Barale, and David M. Halperin, *The Lesbian and Gay Studies Reader* (New York: Routledge, 1993), pp. 397-415.

Schulman, Sarah. *People in Trouble.* New York: Dutton, 1990.

————. *My American History: Lesbian and Gay Life During the Reagan/Bush Years.* New York: Routledge, 1994.

Shilts, Randy. *And the Band Played On: Politics, People, and the AIDS Epidemic.* New York: Penguin, 1988.

————. "Politics Confused With Therapy." *San Francisco Chronicle,* June 26, 1989:A4.

Smith, Dinitia. "The Cry of 'The Normal Heart.'" *New York,* June 3, 1985:42-46.

Span, Paula. "Getting Militant About AIDS." *Washington Post,* March 28, 1989: D1, D4.

Spiers, Herbert R. "AIDS and Civil Disobedience." *Hastings Center Report,* November/December 1989:34-35.

Stacey, Judith. "Can There Be a Feminist Ethnography?" In eds. Sherna Berger Gluck and Daphne Patai, *Women's Words: The Feminist Practice of Oral History* (New York: Routledge, 1991), pp. 111-119.

Staley, Peter. "Has the Direct-Action Group ACT UP Gone Astray?" *Advocate,* July 30, 1991:98.

Treichler, Paula A. "AIDS Narratives on Television: Whose Story?" In eds. Timothy F. Murphy and Suzanne Poirier, *Writing AIDS: Gay Literature, Language, and Analysis* (New York: Columbia University Press, 1993), pp. 161-199.

"United in Anger." *NYQ,* December 8, 1991:26-31.

Vaid, Urvashi. *Virtual Equality: The Mainstreaming of Gay and Lesbian Liberation.* New York: Anchor Books, 1995.

Van Vugt, Johannes P., ed. *AIDS Prevention and Services: Community Based Research.* Westport, CT: Bergin and Garvey, 1994.

Voices from the Front, videotape. Produced by Testing the Limits Collective, 1991.

Watney, Simon. "Political Funeral." *Village Voice,* October 20, 1992:18.

Weales, Gerald. Review of *The Normal Heart,* by Larry Kramer. *Commonweal,* July 12, 1985:406-407.

Weber, Bruce. "'Angels,' Downtown or on Broadway?" *The New York Times,* November 13, 1992:C2.

————."*Angels'* Angels." *New York Times Magazine,* April 25, 1993:29-30, 48-58.

"West Coast Gay Tantrum, The." Editorial. *New York City Tribune,* June 22, 1990.

Winer, Linda. Review of *Millennium Approaches,* by Tony Kushner. *New York Newsday,* May 5, 1993. Reprinted in *New York Theatre Critics' Reviews* 1993:209-210.

————. Review of *Perestroika,* by Tony Kushner. *New York Newsday,* November 24, 1993. Reprinted in *New York Theatre Critics' Reviews* 1993:391.

Winokur, L.A. "I Was Not a Political Animal Before AIDS" (interview with Larry Kramer). *The Progressive,* June 1994:32-35.

Wolfe, Maxine. "The AIDS Coalition to Unleash Power (ACT UP): A Direct Model of Community Research for AIDS Prevention." In ed. Johannes P. Van Vugt, *AIDS Prevention and Services: Community Based Research* (Westport, CT: Bergin and Garvey, 1994), pp. 217-247.

Yang, Jacob Smith. "Activists Protest Inside Capital." *Gay Community News,* October 6-12, 1991:3, 6.

Index

Hammidi, Tania, 13
Hardy, Robin, 130,142-143
Harrington, Mark, 52-54,163n.97
Henry, William A. III, 107-108,113
Heterosexual men
    economic privilege and, 9
    in *People in Trouble*,
        87,91-93,169n.23
Hispanics. *See* People of color
HIV testing, 42-43
Hocking, Peter, 22,56,141
Hoth, Daniel, 52

International Conference on AIDS,
        Sixth (San Francisco), 59,130

Jesdale, Bill, 47-48,57,129,136-137
Johnson, Trina (pseud.),
        50,135,143-144
Jones, Travis (pseud.), 155n.7

Kaiser, Susan, 13
Kayal, Philip, 33-34
Kennedy, Elizabeth Lapovsky,
        146,175n.2,176n.6
Kerrison, Ray, 20
Kraft, Ann (pseud.), 137
Kramer, Larry
    ACT UP/New York and, 33,61
        creation of, 15
    attitudes on sex, 79
    economic privilege and, 81
    GMHC and, 79
    Normal Heart, The
        activism in, 110-112
        celibacy in, 105-107
        crisis of consumption in, 81
        economic privilege in, 83-84,
            168n.17
        form and, 125-126
        Gay Men's Health Crisis
            (GMHC) and, 103,108
        heterosexual audiences
            and, 80-81

Kramer, Larry *(continued)*
    heterosexuals in, 81-84
    individualism in, 112,172n.27
    love story in, 80,103,107-112
    monogamy in, 104-106
    promiscuity in, 106
    sex in, 105-107
Kruger, Steven F., 169n.27
Kushner, Tony
    Angels in America
        awards, 5,170n.4
        Broadway opening of, 5
        closure in, 124-125
        collectivity in, 122-125
        form and, 125-126
        identity politics in, 117
        individualism in, 121-122
        liberalism in, 114-115,117
        love story in, 113-117,119-120
        politics in, 5,113
        production history of,
            170n.3,170n.4
        realism in, 112
        Republicans in, 118-119

Latinos. *See* People of color
Lee, Berna, 32,39-41,160n.67
Leo, John, 20
Lesbian Avengers, The, 58,168n.19
Lesbian and gay studies, 10
Lesbians, in ACT UP/New York,
        18,36-37. *See also* ACT
        UP/New York, women in
Literature and AIDS. *See* AIDS,
        and literature
Love story, 2,101-102. *See also*
        Afterlife, love story in; *Angels
        in America*, love story in;
        Normal Heart, The, love
        story in; *People in Trouble*,
        love story in
    narrative closure and, 102,
        171n.7,171n.8,174n.44
    politics and, 102

For Product Safety Concerns and Information please contact our EU representative GPSR@taylorandfrancis.com Taylor & Francis Verlag GmbH, Kaufingerstraße 24, 80331 München, Germany

T - #0115 - 160425 - C0 - 212/152/11 - PB - 9781560239307 - Gloss Lamination